Höchap

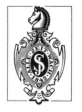

F. Láhoda  A. Ross  W. Issel

# EMG Primer

A Guide to
Practical Electromyography
and Electroneurography

With a Preface by A. Schrader
English Version: J. Payan

With 30 Figures

Springer-Verlag
Berlin Heidelberg New York 1974

Original title of the German edition: "EMG-Fibel", 1973.
Published by Johann Ambrosius Barth, Frankfurt/Main.
ISBN 3-7624-0120-9

Frieder Láhoda, M.D.
Specialist in Internal Medicine, Senior Physician in the Neurological Clinic of the University of Munich, Reader in Neurology at the University of Munich
Neurologische Klinik, D-8 München 70, Marchioninistr. 15

Arno Ross, M.D.
Specialist in Neurology and Psychiatry, Senior Physician in the Neurological Clinic of the University of Munich
Neurologische Klinik, D-8 München 70, Marchioninistr. 15

Walter Issel, M.D.
Specialist in Neurology and Psychiatry, Research Assistant in the Medical Clinic of the University of Erlangen-Nürnberg
Medizinische Klinik und Poliklinik, D-852 Erlangen, Krankenhausstr. 12

The authors wish to extend their thanks to Fred Berninger, engineer in Munich, for preparation of the technical chapter, and to Dr. J. Payan of The National Hospital for Nervous Diseases, Queen's Square, London, for reviewing the English translation.


ISBN 3-540-06992-5 Springer-Verlag Berlin Heidelberg New York
ISBN 0-387-06992-5 Springer-Verlag New York Heidelberg Berlin

This work is subject to copyright. All rights are reserved, whether the whole or part of the material is concerned, specifically those of translation, reprinting, re-use of illustrations, broadcasting, reproduction by photocopying machine or similar means, and storage in data banks.
Under § 54 of the German Copyright Law where copies are made for other than private use, a fee is payable to the publisher, the amount of the fee to be determined by agreement with the publisher. The use of registered names, trademarks, etc. in this publication does not imply, even in the absence of a specific statement, that such names are exempt from the relevant protective laws and regulations and therefore free for general use.

Library of Congress Cataloging in Publication Data
Láhoda, F.
  EMG primer.
  Translation of EMG-Fibel.
  Bibliography: p.
  1. Electromyography. 2. Neuromuscular diseases-Diagnosis. I. Ross, Arno, 1934–    joint author. II. Issel, W., 1940–    joint author. III. Title.
RC77.5.L3313       616.07'54       74-19171
© by Springer-Verlag Berlin · Heidelberg 1974. Printed in Germany.
Composition and Bookbinding by: Appl, Wemding
Printed by: aprinta, Wemding

# Preface to the German Edition

In the last twenty years electromyography and electroneurography have earned a secure position amongst methods of electrophysiological investigation; indeed, it is no longer possible to think of neurological diagnosis without them. In particular, it is in the early recognition of peripheral neuromuscular disorders that these techniques are so dependable and objective. The present text may be thought of as an introduction to method and to diagnostic application, and it should be of value to the physician both in hospital and in his practice. The authors have thought it best to omit discussion of basic scientific problems, which may be found in the neurophysiological literature.

Munich, Spring 1974 A. Schrader

# Contents

| | | |
|---|---|---|
| **1.1** | **Anatomical Foundations** | 1 |
| 1.1.1. | The Motor Unit | 1 |
| 1.1.2. | Structure of the Peripheral Nerve | 1 |
| 1.1.3. | The Neuromuscular Junction | 1 |
| **1.2** | **Electrophysiological Foundations** | 2 |
| 1.2.1. | Origin of Muscle Action Potentials | 2 |
| 1.2.2. | Conduction in the Peripheral Nerve | 3 |
| 1.2.2.1. | Stimulation: Basic Considerations | 3 |
| 1.2.2.2. | Form, Duration and Amplitude of Action Potentials | 4 |
| | a) Evoked Muscle Action Potentials | 4 |
| | b) Nerve and Sensory Action Potentials | 4 |
| | c) Reflex Potentials | 5 |
| **2.1.** | **Technical Foundations** | 5 |
| 2.1.1. | Structure and Function of the Machine | 6 |
| 2.1.1.1. | The Structure of an Electromyograph | 6 |
| 2.1.1.2. | The EMG Amplifier | 7 |
| 2.1.1.3. | Supplementary Measuring Methods in Electromyography | 7 |
| | a) The Stimulator and the Latency Measuring Device | 8 |
| | b) The Delay Line | 9 |
| | c) The Averager | 9 |
| | d) The Digital Averager | 9 |
| **2.2.** | **Electrodes** | 9 |
| 2.2.1. | Main Groups | 10 |
| | a) Electrodes for Action Potential Recording | 10 |
| | b) Electrodes for Stimulation | 10 |
| | c) Earth Electrodes | 10 |
| 2.2.2. | Areas of Use | 10 |
| 2.2.3. | Treatment and Care of Electrodes | 12 |
| **3.1.** | **General Section** | 13 |
| 3.1.1. | The Normal Electromyogram | 13 |
| 3.1.1.1. | Methods of Recording | 13 |
| | a) With Surface Electrodes | 13 |
| | b) With Needle Electrodes | 13 |
| 3.1.1.2. | Procedure in the Electromyographical Examination | 13 |
| 3.1.1.3. | Elements of the Needle Myogram | 15 |

|  |  |  |
|---|---|---|
| | a) Spontaneous Activity | 15 |
| | b) Activity During Voluntary Innervation | 15 |
| 3.1.1.4. | Methods of Registration | 16 |
| | a) Optical | 16 |
| | b) Acoustical | 16 |
| 3.1.2. | The Normal Electroneurogram | 17 |
| 3.1.2.1. | The Motor Electroneurogram | 17 |
| | Stimulation and Recording | 17 |
| | The Normal Examination Procedure | 18 |
| | Registration and Evaluation | 19 |
| 3.1.2.2. | The Sensory Electroneurogram | 20 |
| | The Normal Examination Procedure | 20 |
| | Registration and Evaluation | 21 |
| | The Examination in Children | 22 |
| | Repetitive Stimulation | 23 |
| 3.1.3. | The Pathological Electromyogram | 23 |
| 3.1.3.1. | Lesions of the Lower Motor Neurone | 23 |
| | a) Fasciculation Potentials | 23 |
| | b) Fibrillation Potentials and Positive Sharp Waves | 24 |
| | Pathological Changes in the Pattern on Voluntary Effort | 25 |
| | a) Reduction of the Interference Pattern | 25 |
| | b) Changes in Motor Unit Action Potential Form | 25 |
| | c) Discharge Frequency | 25 |
| 3.1.3.2. | EMG in Primary Muscle Disease | 26 |
| | Spontaneous Activity | 26 |
| | Pathological Changes in the Pattern on Voluntary Effort | 26 |
| | a) Changes in Motor Unit Action Potential Form | 26 |
| | b) Discharge Frequency | 27 |
| 3.1.3.3. | The EMG in Metabolic Electrolyte Disturbances | 27 |
| 3.1.3.4. | The EMG in Centrally-Determined Movement Disturbances | 27 |
| 3.1.4. | The Pathological Electroneurogram | 27 |
| 3.1.4.1. | The Pathological Motor Electroneurogram | 27 |
| 3.1.4.2. | The Pathological Sensory Electroneurogram | 28 |
| 3.1.5. | Disorders of the Neuromuscular Junction | 28 |
| **3.2.** | **Special Section (Diagnosis)** | 29 |
| 3.2.1. | Peripheral Neurogenic Diseases | 30 |
| 3.2.1.1. | General Aspects | 30 |
| 3.2.1.2. | Anterior Horn Cell Diseases | 30 |
| | a) Generalised Anterior Horn Cell Diseases | 31 |
| | b) Local Disorders of Anterior Horn Cells: Poliomyelitis | 32 |

|                |                                                          |    |
|----------------|----------------------------------------------------------|----|
|                | Syringomyelia                                            | 33 |
| 3.2.1.3.       | Root Lesions                                             | 33 |
|                | a) The Intervertebral Disc                               | 33 |
|                | b) Cervical 'Whiplash' Injury                            | 33 |
|                | c) Polyradiculitis (Guillain-Barré)                      | 34 |
|                | d) Other Varieties of Root Lesion                        | 34 |
| 3.2.1.4.       | Plexus Lesions                                           | 34 |
| 3.2.1.5.       | Local Lesions of the Peripheral Nerve                    | 35 |
|                | a) Neuronotmesis                                         | 35 |
|                | b) Axonotmesis                                           | 35 |
|                | c) Neurapraxia                                           | 36 |
|                | d) Reinnervation                                         | 36 |
|                | Compressive Neuropathy                                   | 37 |
|                | a) Carpal Tunnel Syndrome                                | 37 |
|                | b) Cubital Sulcus Syndrome                               | 37 |
|                | c) Chronic Compressive Neuropathies of the Lower Limb    | 38 |
|                | d) Radial Nerve ("Saturday Night Palsy")                 | 38 |
|                | Idiopathic Facial Nerve Palsy (Bell's)                   | 38 |
|                | Trigeminal Neuropathy                                    | 39 |
|                | Polyneuropathies                                         | 39 |
|                | Peroneal Muscular Atrophy                                | 41 |
| 3.2.2.         | Primary Muscle Disease                                   | 41 |
| 3.2.2.1.       | Progressive Muscular Dystrophy (Duchenne)                | 42 |
| 3.2.2.2.       | Inflammatory Muscle Disease (Myositis and Polymyositis)  | 42 |
| 3.2.2.3.       | Late-Onset Myopathies                                    | 43 |
| 3.2.2.4.       | Hereditary Distal Myopathy (Welander)                    | 43 |
| 3.2.2.5.       | Myotonia                                                 | 43 |
| 3.2.3.         | Secondary Myopathies                                     | 44 |
| 3.2.4.         | Myasthenic Syndromes                                     | 44 |
| 3.2.4.1.       | Myasthenia Gravis                                        | 44 |
| 3.2.4.2.       | Symptomatic Myasthenia                                   | 45 |
| 3.2.5.         | Electrolyte Disturbances                                 | 45 |
| 3.2.6.         | Myxoedema                                                | 46 |
| 3.2.7.         | Tetanus                                                  | 46 |
| 3.2.8.         | Centrally-Determined Disturbances of Movement            | 47 |
| 3.2.8.1.       | Spasticity                                               | 47 |
| 3.2.8.2.       | Rigidity                                                 | 47 |
| 3.2.8.3.       | Tremor                                                   | 47 |
|                | a) Rest Tremor in Extrapyramidal Disease                 | 47 |
|                | b) Intention Tremor                                      | 47 |
| 3.2.8.4.       | Torticollis                                              | 48 |

| | | |
|---|---|---|
| 3.2.9. | EMG, ENG and the "Floppy Infant" Syndrome | 48 |
| 3.2.9.1. | Peripheral Neurogenic Lesions | 49 |
| 3.2.9.2. | Myogenic Pareses | 49 |
| 3.2.9.3. | Centrally-Determined Disturbances of Movement | 49 |
| **4.0.** | **EMG of the Extraocular Muscles** | 49 |
| **4.1.** | **Myopathies** | 50 |
| | a) Oligo-Symptomatic Form of Ocular Myositis | 50 |
| | b) Acute Exophthalmic Myositis | 50 |
| | c) Ocular Muscle Dystrophy | 50 |
| | d) Endocrine Ocular Myopathy | 51 |
| | e) Ocular Myotonia | 51 |
| | f) Ocular Myasthenia | 51 |
| **4.2.** | **Peripheral Neurogenic Paresis** | 51 |
| **4.3.** | **Centrally-Determined Disturbances of Movement** | 51 |
| **5.0.** | **Possibilities of Error in the EMG** | 52 |
| **5.1.** | **Possibilities of Error in the ENG** | 52 |
| | a) Motor Electroneurogram | 52 |
| | b) Sensory Electroneurogram | 52 |
| **6.0.** | **Short Introduction to an EMG Examination** | 53 |
| **7.0.** | **Index of Important Terms in Clinical EMG** | 54 |
| **8.0.** | **Index of Important Technical Terms and Abbreviations** | 56 |
| **9.0.** | **Selected Bibliography** | 58 |
| **10.0.** | **Subject Index** | 59 |

# Introduction

The recording of action potentials from muscle, electromyography (hereafter EMG), has become an essential aid in several branches of medicine since the early experiments of the '20s and '30s. It is valuable in diagnosis not only in neurology but in neurosurgery, accident surgery, orthopaedics, internal medicine, paediatrics and ophthalmology. It can be used to distinguish between neurogenic and myogenic pareses, to clarify acute and chronic denervation processes, and to study primary myopathies of degenerative and inflammatory origin, as well as myasthenic syndromes. It is also valuable in the recognition of the disturbance of nerve and muscle function associated with metabolic disease, and in the analysis of centrally-determined movement disorders. Electroneurography is a further refinement, as the function of peripheral nerves may be assessed by means of motor and sensory fibre conduction studies. An important aspect of these techniques is the means they afford of detecting subclinical or latent affection of muscle or nerve, an early appreciation of which is essential in toxic and metabolic disorders. In the same way, regeneration of peripheral nerve is sometimes detectable before clinical recovery.

Until recently the high cost of the complicated apparatus necessary restricted EMG to the larger clinics, but the evolution of equipment has led to widespread and everyday use in keeping with its importance as a diagnostic tool.

Effective use of such equipment demands, as always, familiarity with basic theory, practical experience and an understanding of the diagnostic possibilities. The latter requirement emphasises that EMG differs from EEG and EKG in that it must be performed not by a technician, but by a doctor who has examined the patient clinically.

## 1.1. Anatomical Foundations

A knowledge of certain neuroanatomical facts, briefly indicated below, is indispensable to the practice of EMG and ENG.

### 1.1.1. The Motor Unit

This term is of great importance in EMG, and was coined by Sherrington to describe an anterior horn cell, its axon and all the muscle fibres supplied by it. The number of muscle fibres innervated by a single anterior horn cell varies greatly, the "innervation ratio" in the eye muscles, for example, being 1:5 to 1:10, while in long extremity muscles it may be as much as 1:1500.

### 1.1.2. Structure of the Peripheral Nerve

The gross structure of the nerve is of less importance in the present context than its histology. There are three essential parts: a) the axon cylinder in the centre of the fibre is the extension of the protoplasm of the ganglion cell; b) the myelin sheath which wraps the axon cylinder, and has a varying thickness, is a complicated structure of concentric and radial lipoid and protein lamellae; c) the Schwann cell, lying between each internode, is, with the axon, essential in the formation of the myelin sheath. The peripheral nerve comprises motor, sensory and autonomic fibres.

### 1.1.3. The Neuromuscular Junction

The nerve impulse is not transferred directly to the muscle fibre: a neuromuscular "endplate" is interposed as a chemical synapse, and the junction consists, therefore, of the presynaptic termination of the axon, a synaptic fissure of a few hundred Ångstrom units, and the sub-synaptic membrane of the muscle fibre. As a rule the endplate zone is in the middle of the muscle fibre, only very long fibres having more than one such zone.

## 1.2. Electrophysiological Foundations

The bioelectrical phenomena associated with activity of striped muscle will be given here only as far as is necessary to an understanding of clinical EMG. As already mentioned in the introduction, EMG means the recording, registration and evaluation of muscle action potentials.

### 1.2.1. Origin of Muscle Action Potentials

From the anterior horn cell impulses due to voluntary innervation, or to reflexes, pass by saltatory conduction to the muscle endplate. The time required for this conduction depends fundamentally on the arrangement of the myelin sheath. Since the latter acts as an insulator, the electrical processes basic to stimulus conduction can only occur at the nodes of Ranvier, and this means that the conduction velocity in a myelinated nerve fibre is up to 20 times faster than in an unmyelinated

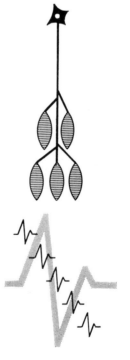

Fig. 1. Diagram of the origin of a motor unit action potential consisting, in this case, of the individual potentials from 5 muscle fibres

fibre of the same diameter. The nerve impulse results in depolarisation at the motor endplate, whence a wave of depolarisation spreads along the fibre membrane with a velocity of 3–4 metres per second (m/sec). This, in turn, leads to activation of the contractile elements and thus to shortening of the muscle fibre.

The bioelectrical correlate of the motor unit consists of the sum of the potentials deriving from individual muscle fibres making up the unit. Variations in form and duration of the 'motor unit action potential' depend partly upon the innervation ratios found in different muscles. The amplitude of a motor unit action potential is greater than the amplitude of a potential from any constituent fibre, due to temporal summation of the small individual potentials; similarly, spatial dispersion of endplate zones explains why contraction of every fibre in a motor unit does not occur simultaneously, and why the motor unit action potential is longer than the potential from any individual fibre.

It should perhaps be mentioned here that electrophysiological stimulation of a muscle through its nerve may be regarded as indirect, while voluntary activation of a muscle is, in this sense, direct or physiological.

## 1.2.2. Conduction in the Peripheral Nerve

*1.2.2.1. Stimulation: Basic Considerations*

In this booklet it is clearly not possible to go into the relevant neurophysiology in detail, and the most important terms will be treated only as key words.

If one applies direct current shocks of increasing intensity to a peripheral nerve or an isolated nerve fibre, an action potential may be recorded once the threshold for stimulation has been exceeded. The size of the current necessary to achieve stimulation, and thus an action potential, is called the threshold current. Currents only just above the threshold will stimulate only a few fibres in the peripheral nerve, and an increasing number of nerve fibres will be "recruited" with increasing current until activation of all fibres results in the total, or "compound", action potential, beyond which no increase in size or change in shape is possible: at this point supramaximal stimulation has been achieved. The all-or-nothing rule applies to single nerve fibres, and these have varying thresholds; it does not apple in a simple manner to the whole peripheral nerve, because the compound action potential is composed of the sum of potentials from individual fibres. Once the nerve has been stimulated, further stimulation is possible only after a short "refractory period", in peripheral nerve about a millisecond, and during this period repolarisation of the membrane takes place. The minimum current which will cause stimulation is called the rheobase, and the time required for a stimulus of twice rheobasic strength to carry the membrane potential to threshold is called the "chronaxie". It is longer in thinner fibres than thicker, and in the case of motor nerves is about 0.1 msec, varying according to size. Chronaximetry, with an exact determination of the threshold value for stimulus strength, is of only minor importance in clinical electrodiagnosis today, but the application of so-called "faradic", short-duration (0.1–1 msec) impulses is as important as ever. These give clearly separated single contractions at about 3/sec, incomplete tetanus from 10/sec and complete tetanus above 50/sec (i.e. a full, sustained contraction of the muscle involved). A tetanus is achieved only by stimulation of the motor nerve, not the muscle directly.

*1.2.2.2. Form, Duration and Amplitude of Action Potentials*

Three main types of potential are under consideration here:

*a) Evoked Muscle Action Potentials.* When the nerve supplying a muscle is stimulated, an evoked action potential is registered in or over the muscle. The time taken from the moment of stimulation to the onset of the potential depends on the distance from the stimulating point to the muscle, and the longer this is, the longer will be the latency. The form and amplitude of the action potential depend largely upon recording conditions. Thus, surface electrodes will show a biphasic potential which is the sum of two monophasic potentials arising under the electrodes (belly-tendon): when the stimulation wave reaches the proximal recording electrode it becomes negative in relation to the distal electrode, and when the distal electrode is reached it, in turn, becomes negative while the proximal electrode is by now positive again. Using bipolar needle electrode recording, or two unipolar needles, the action potentials resemble those recorded with surface electrodes, but need not show a clear biphasic form.

*b) Nerve and Sensory Action Potentials.* When a peripheral mixed nerve is stimulated one may record an action potential from the nerve itself. If the nerve is stimulated at two distal points and a proximal recording is made, one obtains an action potential with a biphasic form. Stimulation of a digit will activate only sensory nerve fibres, and a pure sensory action potential can be recorded over a superficially lying peripheral nerve, e.g. index finger to median nerve at wrist. In certain anatomical situations, e.g. the radial nerve, antidromic stimulation is preferable, but the form of the action potential is similar.

Next to latency, at least at the periphery, the amplitude is the most important parameter in evaluation of the potential (see p. 21).

*c) Reflex Potentials.* When stimulating the peripheral nerve a second muscle action potential is often seen after the directly evoked potential. The latency of this second potential is longer the closer the point of stimulation to the responding muscle, and the explanation for this is assumed to be that the second potential is evoked reflexly via the spinal cord. The latency of this second potential may provide information concerning synaptic delay in the cord, as well as information as to conduction time in afferent and efferent pathways. This reflex potential is called the F wave, and can be obtained by appropriate supramaximal stimulation from the majority of peripheral muscles. A related phenomenon is the H wave, most often seen when the medial popliteal nerve is stimulated in the popliteal fossa and a recording made from the calf muscles. This is essentially the electrophysiological equivalent of the Achilles tendon reflex.

## 2.1. Technical Foundations

A doctor using a piece of technical equipment is interested in the diagnostic help it can give: technical details are usually to him of secondary interest. However, because electrical equipment is designed and built by engineers, its technical features and data have to be expressed in technical terms in order to retain their exact meaning.

It is well known that electric current is measured and expressed in terms of amperes, voltage in volts, and resistance in ohms. However, when advanced electrical measuring equipment is used we find such terms as impedance, conductance, decibel and time constant, which may mean little to the doctor, but which have an essential relevance to the properties of the machine. At the beginning of this technical introduction, therefore, a short explanation will be given in order that something of the structure and function of an EMG machine may be appreciated.

## 2.1.1. Structure and Function of the Machine

Every electronic instrument consists of active and passive parts. Valves, transistors, integrated circuits, certain crystals and diodes, for example, belong to the active parts – active because they have an amplifying function. Passive elements affect electrical qualities by way of signal reduction, examples being rheostats, wiring, condensers, transformers, switches, instruments, regulators etc. All active elements require electrical power; passive networks alone are incapable of functioning when not supplied with some form of energy.

*2.1.1.1. The Structure of an Electromyograph*

The requirements of an instrument used for the examination of nerve and muscle potentials are such that it must consist of a number of systems. In the construction of such a complete measuring instrument both servicing and financial cost must be taken into account, also the exterior shape, size and weight. For ease of use, a logical arrangement of switches, regulators and indicators is essential, and it should be possible to extend the capabilities of the instrument, or to use it in association with other instruments in a more complex system when required. Using the DISA one-channel electromyograph type 14 A 11 as an example, a compact instrument for electromyography is described. It will be useful to look at the block diagram of this instrument.

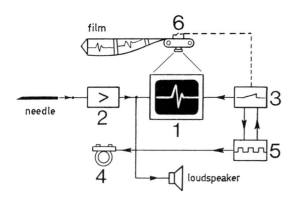

Fig. 2. Block diagram of a DISA one-channel myograph
1 Oscilloscope
2 EMG amplifier
3 Trigger equipment
4 Stimulation electrodes
5 Stimulator
6 Camera

## 2.1.1.2. The EMG Amplifier

The frequency range of the EMG amplifier should be such that all the frequency components of the action potential can be dealt with completely and remain undistorted. Fourier analysis of single action potentials shows a maximum frequency component of approximately 8000 Hz, so an EMG amplifier should have an upper frequency limit of not less than 10,000 Hz to ensure a response free from distortion; the lower frequencies should, similarly, be well within the capacity of the amplifier. The action potentials to be measured are fed through the electrode connection cable to the input socket of the EMG amplifier. The output of the amplifier is connected to the input of a Y amplifier by a socket attachment: this is used to separate the EMG amplifier when, for example, the Y amplifier is used for reproduction from magnetic tape. The Y amplifier produces the necessary output to trigger the oscilloscope. The input of the loudspeaker amplifier is in parallel with the Y amplifier, which makes the action potentials audible through a built-in or externally connected loudspeaker. The output of a sweep generator is fed to the horizontal deflection plates of the cathode ray tube through the X amplifier. The X sweep is triggered by the impulse generator, which in turn is activated either by the trigger generator or by an external trigger signal. A stimulus indicator is locked directly to the impulse generator; this triggers the stimulus generator, which allows control of frequency and amplitude of the stimulus pulse. This pulse is delivered through an output transformer, and in addition triggers the digital indicator for the latency of the response.

A chopper amplifier can be installed as an additional device. This turns the machine into a two-beam machine, the second beam then serving as a DC input for the connection of additional measuring devices such as averagers, muscle thermometers and so on. Signals shown on the screen may be recorded with a polaroid camera set. In this way the amplification and sweep speed are automatically shown by two digital indicators on the right and left side of the photograph.

## 2.1.1.3. Supplementary Measuring Methods for Electromyography

Besides showing muscle and nerve action potentials, myographs can be fitted with devices to give additional information. The one-channel electromyograph is automatically furnished with one of these additional devices:

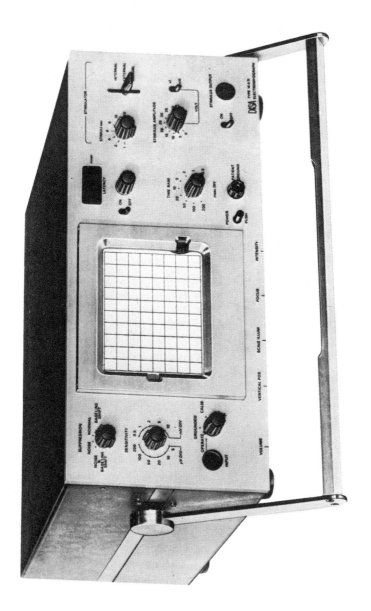

Fig. 3. Portable one-channel myograph (Disa Electronics A/S Herlev, Denmark)

*a) The Stimulator and the Latency Measuring Device.* For the investigation of responses to electrical stimuli a stimulator suitable to both muscle and nerve is used. Square wave impulses of variable width and height have proved suitable used singly or in a train. Stimulus artefact is visible on the screen, always at the same place on the left side. This is in order to measure the reaction time following a stimulus impulse: latencies between stimulus and response allow calculation of nerve conduction velocity (see p. 20). A nomogram makes possible direct reading of the conduction velocity. Trains of impulses are necessary for the investigation of myasthenia. These may be given at different frequencies and may be of different duration. The stimulus width can be set at from 0.05 to 1 msec, and the frequency at from 1 to 100 Hz. The voltage can be varied from 0 to 500 volts.

*b) The Delay Line.* When the sweep of the oscilloscope is triggered by the action potential, randomly occurring action potentials can be made to appear at a constant position on the screen. To avoid losing the initial phase of the potential a delay line is used, which postpones the appearance of the action potential and allows the entire potential to be made visible.

*c) The Averager.* When direct measurement of muscle tension cannot be made, mechanical activity can be fairly exactly estimated by integrating electrical activity: experiments on isometrically contracting muscles show that the integral value of the electromyogram is proportional to the simultaneously registered muscle tension. The averager possesses two similar integrators with a time constant of 50 msec, a suitable value giving a curve smooth enough but still fast enough to follow changes.

*d) The Digital Averager.* Small evoked potentials are difficult to demonstrate when interfered with by larger, randomly occurring potentials, as is almost always the case with sensory potentials. The averager increases the signal/noise ratio by adding, and thus averaging out, unwanted random interference.

## 2.2. Electrodes

Electrodes used for recording action potentials are chosen for the purpose intended, and there is available a range of electrodes which meet all the above-mentioned technical requirements; it comprises the following main groups:

## 2.2.1. Main Groups

   a) Electrodes for action potential recording
   b) Electrodes for stimulation
   c) Earth electrodes

Within these groups are the following subdivisions:
   for recording and stimulating:
      Surface electrodes
      Bipolar needle electrodes
      Multielectrodes
      Teflon-covered electrodes
      Implantable electrodes
   for recording:
      Concentric needle electrodes
      Oesophageal electrodes
      Catheter electrodes
   for stimulation:
      Nerve root electrodes


## 2.2.2. Areas of Use

The following is a review of the application of these various electrodes. Surface electrodes are used mainly for stimulation, and usually consist of felt pads. They may be hand-held or fastened securely to the skin overlying the nerve with a strap. Surface electrodes may also be used for monitoring the activity of agonists and antagonists, as well as for evaluating more gross activity. Concentric needle electrodes are steel tubes with platinum cores, the whole of which is embedded in araldite. They have varying diameters, lengths and plugs. The muscle action potentials are picked up between the platinum surface and the tube, the latter acting as the indifferent electrode. The electrodes are connected to the amplifier socket by shielded two-lead cable. For very small muscles, e.g. extraocular, a special thin electrode of only 0.3 mm diameter (type 13 K 59/or 13 L 58) is generally used. The platinum core of these types has a surface area of only 0.15 mm$^2$.

Bipolar needle electrodes possessing two platinum cores with especially small surfaces are used for simultaneous registration of several motor units, and for local stimulation of nerve and muscle.

Multi-electrodes are used for the determination of motor unit territory, but may also be used for stimulation.

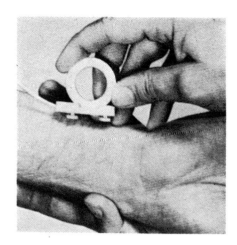

Fig. 4. Commercial stimulation electrode

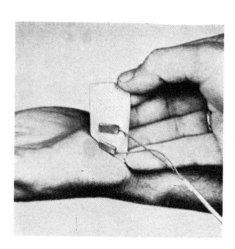

Fig. 5. Commercial bi-polar surface electrode such as is used for
a) registration of the total activity of a muscle or
b) registration of the responses to stimulation during neurography

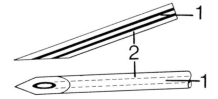

Fig. 6. Diagram of a concentric needle electrode
1 Platinum core
2 Steel casing

Teflon-convered electrodes are isolated steel electrodes whose 3–5 mm long tips are uncovered. These were specially developed for recording sensory action potentials, and can only be used in conjunction with pre-amplifiers for the registration of nerve action potentials. In order to record what are often very small potentials (about 1 µv) the electrode should be galvanically treated before every examination.

Oesophageal electrodes are used for registering the muscle activity of the diaphragm. The electrode is inserted through the nose into the oesophagus as far as the top of the diaphragm. Catheter electrodes are used for examination of sphincter and bladder musculature.

Nerve root electrodes were developed for recording from nerves exposed during operations.

Implantable electrodes are used mainly for studies of movement: since the platinum wires are very flexible they scarcely hinder the muscle's freedom of movement.

Earth electrodes are used to ensure that the patient is at neutral potential in order to prevent electrical interference from the immediate environment. They are also used as a means of diminishing stimulus artefact, and for this purpose are placed at a point between the stimulating and the recording electrodes.

### 2.2.3. Treatment and Care of Electrodes

Only when needle electrodes are properly sharpened can they be inserted comparatively painlessly. The point of the tube should be ground to an angle of 15–20° in order to guarantee a surface of 0.07 mm$^2$ at the platinum core tip. The point should also be diagonally ground at the side in order to create a kind of trochar form (see Fig. 6). Grinding should be done with a fine sand paper, and the electrode should be inspected to make sure it is isolated from the steel casing; this is especially important with very thin electrodes. The electrode must be treated electrolytically after grinding. This can be done with the power generator which is supplied as an attachment for sensory nerve measurements, or with a 6 V transformer with alternating current, or else with a battery and direct current. The electrode is lowered into a glass vessel containing physiological saline (0.9%), and the current source is connected between the platinum electrode and the tube connections. The current is allowed to flow for 1–2 seconds, or until one or two gas bubbles detach themselves from the surface of the platinum electrode. In order to avoid irreparable damage to the platinum surface this process should not last longer than stated. The galvanic procedure markedly reduces electrode impedance, and noise is lowered to less than 15 µv.

## 3.1. General Section

### 3.1.1. The Normal Electromyogram

*3.1.1.1. Methods of Recording*

*a) With Surface Electrodes:* A record taken with surface electrodes gives only a general impression of the electrical activity of whole muscle groups or, less often, individual muscles. It may, however, be useful in the investigation of central distrubances of innervation and in mechanomyography.

*b) With Needle Electrodes:* By contrast, recording with a needle inserted in the muscle provides exact and detailed information concerning individual motor unit action potentials, and hence the functional state of the lower motor neurone. The most important application of this is, of course, the differentiation of myopathic and neurogenic disorders. The dimensions of the needle in relation to those of the muscle fibre mean that recording is always extracellular, the potentials being either spontaneous or the result of voluntary activation of the muscle.

*3.1.1.2. Procedure in the Electromyographical Examination*

There is no fixed procedure in the plan of an electromyographical investigation; its form, unlike some other electrophysiological investigations, depends not only upon the clinical problem under consideration but also upon information gained in the course of it, and a knowledge of peripheral anatomy, especially of innervation, is indispensable. The investigation should be performed in a comfortably warm room so that the patient may be undressed without shivering – a source of artefact. An examination couch is necessary so that the patient can lie, usually on his back, in as relaxed a position as possible; adequate cushioning should be available so that he can be equally comfortable on his stomach when paravertebral muscles are to be investigated. Account should be taken of the common unspoken fear among patients of "electricity", and an explanation given that muscle sampling is comparable to recording an EKG.
Each investigation demands a sharp needle sterilised, according to type, by autoclave or immersion in formaldehyde vapour. Analgesic and local anesthetic drugs are not necessary, though in some anxious patients

mild sedation is often helpful. Few patients find the investigation too painful to tolerate, and it is unusual to have to terminate it on this account. An adequate investigation may be difficult in children, mainly because they are unable or unwilling to activate a muscle weakly enough to allow analysis of single motor unit action potentials. When this is the case it is often helpful to employ reflex activation of the muscle; for example, tibialis anterior will contract in response to stroking the sole of the foot. There are, in general, no absolute contra-indications to needle myography, though particular care must obviously be taken when investigating muscles such as serratus anterior and trapezius. A relative contra-indication may be held to exist when the patient is on anticoagulants, and in situations where infection would be particularly undesirable, such as diabetes mellitus and local skin disorders. If the doctor performing the investigation has not already examined the patient clinically he must do so before embarking upon electromyography. In particular, he must test the power of muscles he intends to sample before inserting the needle as pain may then discourage a maximal effort. The patient can then be shown how he will be required to contract the muscles concerned after the needle has been inserted. It is usual to begin with a clinically normal muscle. The entry of the needle will be heard rather than seen and any insertion activity will last little longer than the movement of the needle; the presence of insertion activity indicates that the tip of the needle has entered the muscle proper. The loudspeaker should have been switched on before insertion of the needle so that no early potentials of any kind are missed. Then, with the muscle completely relaxed, the investigator watches and listens for spontaneous activity. So-called endplate noise can be distinguished from short duration potentials of pathological significance by its form and by the ease with which readjustment of the needle position will abolish it. When a healthy muscle is relaxed no action potentials should be registered, but this is not the case with extra-ocular muscles, which always show some basic continuous activity (stabilisation of the eye). Having ascertained that there is no spontaneous activity, the patient is now asked to activate the muscle; one can start with a maximal effort, but it is more usual to ask for the weakest possible contraction in order to study individual motor unit action potentials. The number of units observed may be increased by moving the needle vertically and thus sampling several different sites, using auditory information to determine optimal positions of the tip. Recruitment of further potentials and increase in discharge frequency can then be achieved by asking the patient to progressively increase his effort; this results eventually in the interference pattern.

## 3.1.1.3. Elements of the Needle Myogram

a) Spontaneous activity
b) Activity during voluntary innervation

*a) Spontaneous activity* in normal muscle comprises insertion activity and end-plate noise. The first consists of a brief discharge of usually low-voltage potentials lasting only a little longer than the movement of the needle, and is therefore more easily heard than seen. These potentials arise not from whole motor units, but probably from mechanical damage to one or several muscle fibres; they may thus recur when the needle is moved. End-plate noise occurs when the needle tip lies in the end-plate zone of the muscle, and consists of a high frequency discharge of short-duration, low-voltage potentials which generally lasts longer than insertion activity. End-plate noise is interpreted as either extracellularly recorded miniature end-plate potentials or mechanically discharged intramuscular nerve action potentials.

*b) Voluntary Activity.* A needle in striated muscle picks up potentials from 4–6 motor units during voluntary activation. These units are recruited successively with increasing effort, and at the same time the discharge frequency (i.e. the firing rate of each respective motor unit) increases to a degree determined by the force the muscle is required to exert. This discharge frequency begins at about 1/sec and may increase to more than 100/sec. Even medium strength activation will result in motor unit action potentials running into each other, so that the base-

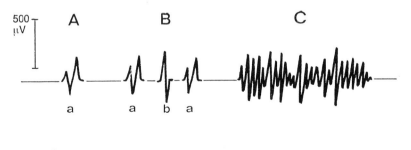

Fig. 7. The origin of the interference pattern
A: A single motor unit (a) discharges during weak voluntary effort
B: The unit fires during increasing effort and a second unit (b) is recruited
C: Interference activity; single units can no longer be distinguished one from another

line disappears and individual potentials can no longer be distinguished, the so-called "interference pattern".

Thus, only with weak effort can individual motor unit action potentials be studied with regard to form, duration and amplitude.

As discussed under 1.2, the form of the action potential in a given muscle is related to the number of muscle fibres in each motor unit and their spatial distribution; the largest amplitudes are met where the proportion of anterior horn cells to muscle fibres is high, as, for example, in small hand muscles. The largest mean motor unit "territory" is found in muscles such as rectus femoris and extensor digitorum longus, and the smallest in the external ocular muscles, where an arrangement of 5–10 muscle fibres per unit makes fine control possible. Normal motor unit action potentials tend to have two to three and sometimes four phases, and when there are more than four the potential is described as polyphasic; only a small percentage of potentials are polyphasic in a healthy muscle. The mean duration of normal motor unit action potentials is 5–15 msec, and the amplitude varies from 200–2000 μV), depending on the distance of the needle tip from the motor unit. In older age groups, or with a fall in muscle temperature, or if the patient is tired, the potential duration tends to be longer and associated with polyphasia; this is probably due to a reduction in conduction velocity in terminal nerve fibres leading to increased desynchronisation within the motor unit.

### 3.1.1.4. Methods of Registration

*a) Optical.* Because of the relatively high frequencies concerned, mechanical writing systems are generally unsuitable in electromyography, and the cathode ray oscilloscope is used.

*b) Acoustical.* The capacity of the human ear for distinguishing certain frequencies is so great that it is very important to hear as well as see the amplified signals being picked up by the needle, and they should be relayed through a loudspeaker simultaneously with their appearance on the oscilloscope screen.

Potentials of pathological significance may, by this means, be picked up by ear alone.

### 3.1.2. The Normal Electroneurogram

*3.1.2.1. The Motor Electroneurogram*

*Stimulation and Recording*

A distinction has already been made between electrodes for stimulation and for recording (see p. 10). When surface electrodes are used for either purpose the surrounding skin must be carefully cleaned, and in order to improve electrical conductivity the anode and cathode are smeared with an electrical paste which is in normal commercial use. In routine examination for motor nerve conduction velocity the following areas are commonly used for positioning the stimulating electrode: arm- Erb's point, axilla, at elbow, at wrist (Fig. 8) and

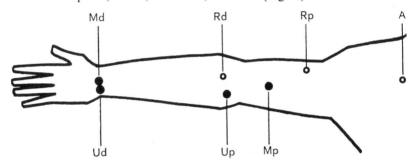

Fig. 8. diagram of the usual points of stimulation along the arm
Ud Distal ulnar, Up Proximal ulnar, Md Distal median, Mp Proximal median, Rd Distal radial (outer side of arm), Rp Proximal radial (outer side of arm), A Axilla; additional point for proximal stimulation of ulnar nerve

leg- popliteal fossa, at ankle (Fig. 9).

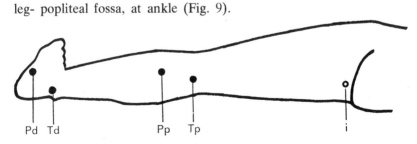

Fig. 9. Diagram of the usual points of stimulation along the leg
Pd Distal peroneal, Pp Proximal peroneal, Td Distal tibial, Tp Proximal tibial, I Sciatic

The determination of motor conduction velocity in nerves such as the radial, sciatic and femoral is more difficult than in more superficially placed nerves.

Either concentric needle electrodes or surface electrodes may be used for recording evoked muscle action potentials, placed either directly over the muscle belly or inserted into it. Unipolar or bipolar needles may be used. The most widely used muscles for the determination of motor nerve conduction velocity are the following:

Table 1. Muscles usually employed in determining motor conduction velocity

| | |
|---|---|
| Ulnar nerve – | Abductor digiti minimi, 1st dorsal interosseus |
| Median nerve – | Abductor pollicis brevis, opponens pollicis |
| Lateral popliteal nerve – | Extensor digitorum brevis |
| Medial popliteal (tibial) nerve – | Flexor hallucis brevis |
| Sciatic nerve – | Extensor digitorum brevis or flexor hallucis br. |

*The Normal Examination Procedure*

When the various electrodes are in place the method can be briefly demonstrated to the patient by giving him some stimuli so as to accustom him to what he may find uncomfortable. He should be told that he can make a great contribution to the success of the examination by relaxing as completely as possible. He should be taught that silence from the loudspeaker is indicative of complete relaxation. Stimulation may begin as soon as the investigator is confident that electrodes are in the optimal position. A short duration (0.1 msec) stimulus is usually used, at least initially, and the stimulus strength increased from threshold to supramaximal. The form, amplitude and latency of the evoked potential may be followed on the screen.

*When the shape and latency of the potential do not change with increasing current strength, then all nerve fibres have been recruited by the stimulus, which is of supramaximal strength.*

The use of different strengths of stimulus between threshold and supramaximal will demonstrate that potentials of differing latency can be evoked according to the presence of nerve fibres with different conduction velocities.

Electroneurographical examinations should always be carried out at an even room temperature and, when possible, humidity. The skin temperature should be at least 34° overlying the muscle being examined, and the possibility of cooling during the investigation remembered: a reduction of skin temperature by 1° may reduce nerve conduction velocity by 2.4 m/sec.

In order to keep stimulus artefact to a minimum the earth electrode should be placed between the stimulating and the recording electrodes. To obtain a clear and unequivocal initial deflection from the base-line ("take-off") as the point of onset of the potential it is essential that:

1. Stimulating electrodes lie as close as possible to the nerve,
2. The stimulating cathode is always distal.

*Registration and Evaluation*

The normal motor electroneurogram consists of stimulus artefact, latency and evoked muscle action potential. The form and amplitude of the potential may vary, but under proper conditions it should be clear and artefact-free, with a sharp onset and a smooth course. Precise measurement of distal and proximal latencies is essential for calculation of an accurate conduction velocity.

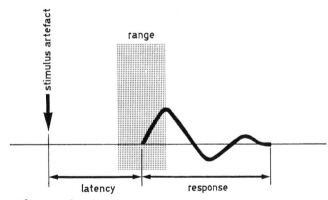

Fig. 10. Diagram of a normal motor electroneurogram

With some instruments it is possible to determine latency and amplitude of response directly from the oscilloscope, but otherwise measurements have to be made from a photograph. If one has obtained the latencies to a muscle from two different stimulating points, one distal and one proximal, a knowledge of the distance between these two points will enable a conduction velocity to be calculated. The following example is intended to demonstrate this: the distance from the cathode over the median nerve in the cubital fossa to that over the nerve at the wrist is 24 cm; the distal latency is 4 msee and the proximal latency 8 msec, the difference being 4 msec; then the motor nerve conduction velocity is 60 m/sec, according to the formular:

$$\text{Motor conduction velocity (m/sec)} = \frac{\text{Distance (mm)}}{\text{Proximal-distal latency (msec)}}$$

Motor conduction velocity is commonly faster in the upper than in the lower extremities, and in proximal segments of nerve than distal, the latter because the myelin sheath is thicker proximally. Normal values for conduction velocity in individual nerves differ somewhat according to the apparatus and techniques used, so it is desirable that a set of normal values be established in each laboratory. As a guide, however, the following values are used in our own laboratory.

Table 2. Normal values

| |
|---|
| Median nerve – cubital fossa to wrist 46–72 m/sec; mean 57 |
| Ulnar nerve – cubital fossa to wrist 47–72 m/sec; mean 60 |
| Medial popliteal nerve – knee to ankle 40–67 m/sec; mean 50 |
| Lateral popliteal nerve – knee to ankle 42–63 m/sec; mean 52 |

These values indicate the normal range.

### 3.1.2.2. The Sensory Electroneurogram

For stimulation ring electrodes are used, and for recording surface or needle electrodes (see p. 10).

*The Normal Examination Procedure*

Though a little more complicated than the determination of motor conduction velocity, the orthodromic sensory neurogram of the median and ulnar nerves is similar in principle and relatively easy. Ring electrodes are placed on the appropriate fingers, one over the distal and one over the proximal phalanx. The distal ring electrode acts as anode and the proximal as cathode. Recording electrodes are applied to the wrist and elbow areas according to the nerve being investigated. Attention should be paid to the moistening of the ring electrodes with saline or jelly, the previous preparation of the skin with alcohol or ether, and the prevention of a bridge of moisture or jelly between the electrodes. Skin resistance can be determined at this stage, and if it is particularly greasy the skin can be abraided with pumice stone.

If the ulnar nerve is to be stimulated the ring electrodes are placed on the little finger, and the recording electrodes anywhere along the course of the nerve up to the level of the axilla. In the case of the median nerve, the index finger may be stimulated and recording made from wrist to above elbow. The recording of an orthodromic action potential from the radial nerve is more difficult, so antidromic recording is often used. Orthodrimic recording is easier from the lateral popliteal nerve, the point of stimulation being at the anterior aspect of the ankle, and of recording at the head of the fibula. In this case it is better to use fine needles inserted near the nerve along its course, with an interelectrode distance of ca. 4 cm. Sensory electroneurography differs from motor in that high amplification is always necessary. As in motor ENG it is important that the stimulating and recording electrodes lie as close as possible to the nerve, but the stimulating cathode is proximal.

*Registration and Evaluation*

In the sensory ENG the latency, amplitude and form of the potential have to be considered. Because of the difficulty of discriminating the precise onset of the potential from noise, it is often necessary to measure latency to the first negative peak of the potential; clearly, if this measurement "to peak" is used, it must be used for both proximal and distal stimulating points. If, when attempting to measure sensory conduction velocity, a potential is so small as to be lost in noise, two fingers may be stimulated simultaneously with separate but synchronised stimulators. Other methods of producing a potential large enough to be distinguished from noise are a) photographic superposition of repeated sweeps, and b) with storage oscilloscope or electronic digital averager. The amplitude of the sensory action potential in normal subjects depends very much on details of technique. It is calculated by comparing the peak to peak distance in mm with the height of a known calibration signal, e.g. 10 $\mu v$ = 10 mm. Potentials recorded distally usually lie between 8 and 20 $\mu v$, while proximally recorded potentials are usually

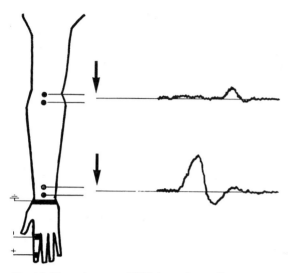

Fig. 11. Normal sensory ENG from the median nerve

of less than 10 µv. Valuable information as to the pathological nature of a lesion may be gained by considering the amplitude of a sensory action potential (or mixed nerve AP) in relation to its latency.

Table 3. Average values of distal sensory latencies

| | |
|---|---|
| Wrist | median nerve: 2.5–4 msec |
| | ulnar nerve: 2.5–4 msec |
| Elbow | median nerve: 6–8 msec |
| | ulnar nerve: 6–8 msec |
| Ankle | lateral popliteal nerve: 4–5 msec |
| Capitulum fibulae | lateral popliteal nerve: 8–11 msec |

Whether a potential is measured to its apparent onset or "to peak" should always be recorded.

*The Examination in Children*

This may not even be possible, in view of the importance of relaxation in sensory recording, but if the child can be calmed sufficiently to make it worthwhile starting, it is at least advisable to avoid using needle electrodes. Surface electrodes should be of appropriately small size, with respect to surface area and cathode – anode distance; a reduction by 40–50% has been found adequate. If needle electrodes simply cannot be avoided then a local anaesthetic such as 2% novocaine may be helpful, bearing in mind that a risk of altering the ENG then arises.

*Repetitive Stimulation*

A knowledge of the technique of repetitive stimulation is essential for the study of myasthenia. Surface recording over hypothenar muscles and stimulation of the ulnar nerve at the wrist is a commonly employed method. Intramuscular needle recording tends to introduce artefact due to needle movement, and stimulating the median nerve is often more painful than the ulnar. Frequency of stimulation is usually between 1 and 50 /sec (see p. 44).

### 3.1.3. The Pathological Electromyogram

*3.1.3.1. Lesions of the Lower Motor Neurone*

Lesions of the lower motor neurone are characterised by spontaneous activity and by changes in the pattern on voluntary effort. Spontaneous activity is of the following kinds:

*a) Fasciculation Potentials.* This is the spontaneous firing of one or several motor units, and indicates hyper-irritability of the lower motor neurone. In Wallerian degeneration it may occur until the process has reached the motor endplate, when the functional unit is of course disrupted. Although the exact mode of origin is not known, fasciculation may be found in lesions of any part of the lower motor neurone, particularly anterior horn cell and nerve root. The form, duration and amplitude of a fasciculation potential are as variable as in the case of ordinary motor unit action potentials, and depend on the extent to which the unit has already been affected. In so called "benign" fasciculation, the appearance may be that of a normal unit, and reflects merely a state of hyper-irritability. In fact even "malign" fasciculations may have the appearance of normal units, and since there is no sure way of knowing the significance of a fasciculation from the point of view of pathology, it should be considered only in the context of the other electromyographical findings. This said, however, it is true that anterior horn cell disease is the most common cause of pathological fasciculation, when randomly occuring discharges of variable but usually low frequency are seen. One hears a full, rather muffled sound, seeming to come from further away than is the actual case, and the amplitude is usually more than 4 mV. Fasciculation occurring near the surface of the muscle can often be seen through the skin as a flickering or twitching over a small area, but those fasciculations arising deeply in the muscle are naturally accessible only to the exploring needle.

*b) Fibrillation Potentials and Positive Sharp Waves.* In contrast to fasciculation, fibrillation is never visible to the naked eye except in the tongue. It will arise when a denervation process has reached the endplate region, consequent changes in muscle membrane potential now rendering the fibre sensitive to much smaller quantities of transmitter substance than normal. The spontaneous release of small packets of acetylcholine at the nerve terminal results in muscle fibre contraction even in the absence of a centrally-originating nerve impulse. Every change in position of the needle may give a shower of fibrillation potentials which fade within minutes, usually with diminishing frequency; they generally have a rhythmic character, and, representing contraction of individual muscle fibres, have correspondingly small spikelike forms with one or two phases. The duration of an individual fibrillation is seldom more than 1.5–2 msec, but the amplitude varies, according to the size of the fibre and the position of the recording needle, up to 100 μV in most cases. The discharge frequency is between 2–5 and 30/sec. A less common spontaneous potential of short duration is the positive sharp wave which, as its name implies, has an initial downward deflection from the base line. The amplitude and duration of the positive sharp wave vary more than do those of the fibrillation potential.

Both types of potential suggest still-active denervation processes, hence the term "denervation potentials", but they are by no means pathognomonic of a lower motor neurone lesion as they can occur in other conditions involving a morphological or functional alteration of muscle fibre membrane potential, for example myositis (see p. 42). In denervation processes of long standing, spontaneous activity may be seen in the form of a high frequency discharge, the "pseudomyotonic" discharge, to be differentiated from the true myotonic discharge by the ease with which the latter may be evoked by percussion of the muscle (see p. 43).

## Pathological Changes in the Pattern on Voluntary Effort

*a) Reduction of the Interference Pattern.* In neurogenic lesions whole motor units drop out, in contrast to myopathies. According to the extent to which motor units are lost, the interference pattern will become rarefied on maximal voluntary effort, until, when only one or two units remain, the pattern is no longer one of interference but one of discrete activity. In this case the single units can be seen to be firing with increased frequency.

*b) Changes in Motor Unit Action Potential Form.* The single most important way in which the organism attempts to compensate for loss of motor units is by peripheral sprouting, in which healthy and intact motor units take over responsiblity for innervating muscle fibres which have lost their nerve supply. The necessary sprouting of terminal nerve fibres from healthy nerves extends their territory, and this in turn increases the duration of the resulting potential. The incorporation of denervated muscle fibres into a healthy motor unit tends to increase not only the duration but the number of phases, and hence the complexity, of the motor unit potential.

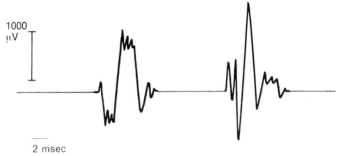

Fig. 12. Neurogenic reconstruction, showing motor unit action potentials of increased duration, amplitude (c. 2000 µV) and number of phases

*c) Discharge Frequency.* The second means of compensating for loss of motor units is to increase the rate of firing of surviving motor units above their usual discharge frequency. Less important diagnostically than the above changes in form, this nevertheless contributes to the picture of the neurogenic lesion.

## 3.1.3.2. EMG in Primary Muscle Disease

After muscle biopsy, EMG is the most important means of detecting and observing primary muscle disease. Here the muscle fibre is involved primarily, and not secondarily through a lesion of its nerve supply. EMG findings indicate myopathy but not, however, the nature of the pathological process responsible, with the possible exception of myotonic dystrophy (see under 43).

### Spontaneous Activity

Spontaneous activity in primary myopathy is unusual except in the advanced stages, when fibrillation potentials indicate persistent membrane damage.

### Pathological Changes in the Pattern on Voluntary Effort

*a) Changes in Motor Unit Action Potential Form.* The form, duration and amplitude of potentials in primary myopathies differ markedly from the findings in neuropathies. In the former, the atrophy and loss of individual fibres results in a diminished number of muscle fibres per motor unit, and hence to a shortening of the motor unit potential, and

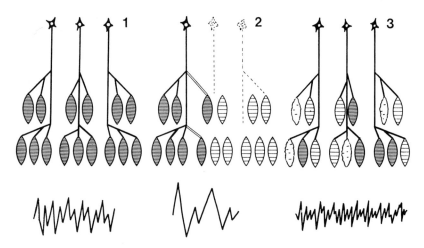

Fig. 13. The pattern on maximal voluntary activity. 1 Normal interference pattern, 2 Peripheral neurogenic lesion (double line = collateral sprouting), 3 Myopathy

a reduction in its amplitude. The drop-out of muscle fibres from the units also results in a polyphasic appearance, possibly related to a disturbance in the spread of excitation along the fibre membrane.

*b) Discharge Frequency.* A further indication of the presence of a primary myopathy is the attempted compensation for weakness by early recruitment of all available motor units, resulting in an apparent discrepancy between weakness of actual movement and density of interference pattern.

### 3.1.3.3. The EMG in Metabolic Electrolyte Disturbances

In metabolic electrolyte disturbances rhythmical multiple discharges may occur spontaneously or on appropriate provocation. Fibrillation potentials are also occasionally seen, but the pattern on effort remains unchanged generally. Pressure by means of a sphygmomanometer cuff around the upper arm, applied while the patient is hyperventilating for 3–5 minutes, will usually provoke these multiple discharges, but not everyone can hyperventilate vigorously for as long as this. Recording is best made with fine needles in the first dorsal interosseus.

### 3.1.3.4. The EMG in Centrally-Determined Movement Disturbances

Simultaneous recording from agonists and antagonists, using a multichannel electromyograph, may reveal valuable information on both voluntary and reflex activation. Clinically latent activity may be demonstrated by means of a concentric needle electrode during passive extension of a muscle, making possible differentiation between spasticity, rigidity and tremor. A quantitative analysis is possible when a clinically overt stage has been reached.

### 3.1.4. The Pathological Electroneurogram

#### 3.1.4.1. The Pathological Motor Electroneurogram

Provided that one or more motor units are still supplied by an intact nerve, a muscle action potential can be evoked by stimulation of that nerve, but the form, duration and amplitude of the potential will be related to the severity of the damage to the nerve. Although, especially in polyneuropathies, the distal motor latency is often increased, the presence of a single normal fast-conducting fibre will result in a normal latency. A reduction on motor conduction velocity is a valuable finding, but the existence of a fairly wide normal range must be borne in mind.

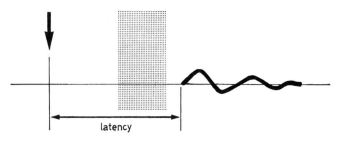

Fig. 14. Diagram of the pathological motor electroneurogram. Increase in latency (combined with changing potential form of the response)

### 3.1.4.2. *The Pathological Sensory Electroneurogram*

An increase in latency is, again, the single most important pathological change, but a reduction in amplitude, especially to less than 10 μV, may be taken as an indication of damage to the nerve, whether of mechanical, toxic, metabolic or other cause.

### 3.1.5. Disorders of the Neuromuscular Junction

Transmission at the motor endplate is by means of the discharge of transmitter material from nerve endings depolarising the endplate zone and causing muscle contraction. Disorders of this region may involve primarily the nerve endings or the endplate itself, and may arise:

a) During the build-up of transmitter material
b) During the discharge of transmitter material
c) By competitive inhibition; other substances occupy the sites of action of the transmitter material on the endplate
d) By suppression due to hyperpolarisation; this may result from excess of cholinesterase or high concentration of acetylcholine

In the case of the best known disorder in this region, myasthenia gravis, the mechanism of the disturbance has not yet been fully worked out, though the effect of physostigmine, prostigmin, mestinon and other substances has been used therapeutically for years. Repetitive stimulation plays an important role in the diagnosis of myasthenia. Often a clue may have been provided by fluctuation and sometimes disappearance of a potential during needle recording, but the use of trains of supramaximal stimuli at various frequencies, e.g. 2, 5, 10, 20, 30, 40, 50/sec results in the myasthenic patient in a typical fall-off in amplitude of the muscle response without recovery, unlike the results in normal subjects, where unsystematic fluctuations in amplitude occur. (For the means of differentiating between myasthenia gravis and other causes of myasthenia, see p. 45).

## 3.2. Special Section (Diagnosis)

Here we shall consider those diseases in which EMG and ENG are especially helpful. A semi-diagrammatic picture is drawn from original polaroid photographs, and in the majority of cases the pathological EMG examples have the normal pattern as a background (Fig. 15).

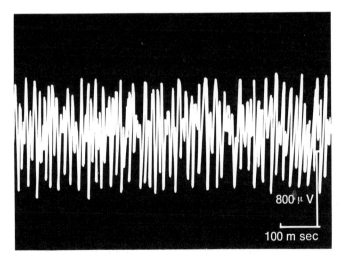

Fig. 15. Normal interference pattern (partly diagrammatic). For comparison this normal curve is projected on to most of the pathological examples (also partly diagrammatic). Unless special mention is made, all patterns have the same calibration and sweep speed

### 3.2.1. Peripheral Neurogenic Diseases

*3.2.1.1. General Aspects*

Paralysis is found only when damage to a nerve is of fairly severe degree, but clinically latent damage may be readily revealed by means of EMG and ENG. Further, when lesions are severe these techniques can demonstrate that denervation is either total or subtotal: from the clinical point of view such differentiation may not be possible, since there is a limit to the compensation which a few undamaged fibres can achieve. The following questions can usually be answered by means of EMG and ENG:
  Is the injury local, or is there a generalised affection?
  Is it the plexus or the distal part of the nerve which is affected?
  Is the damage of acute or chronic nature?
  What evidence is there of regeneration?


*3.2.1.2. Anterior Horn Cell Diseases*

Anterior horn cell disease results in the loss of whole motor units, and the organism attempts to compensate for this by collateral sprouting of healthy units in the neighbourhood of damaged ones. The latter process results in changes in potential duration, maximum amplitude and incidence of polyphasia which are often of much greater degree than is the case in more peripheral lesions; so-called "giant potentials" have maximum amplitudes of over 4 and as much as 15 mV. According to the acuteness of the disease spontaneous activity will be more or less prominent, and according to the severity of the motor unit loss the rarefaction of the interference pattern and the increase in firing rate already described will also occur to varying degrees.
Fasciculation is a particularly important aspect of the spontaneous activity occurring in anterior horn cell disease. Since only the anterior horn cell is damaged, moreover, the conduction velocity in the peripheral nerve is not significantly affected, providing a point of contrast with more distal lesions. Few normally conducting fibres need survive for a normal conduction velocity to be present, as already mentioned. The EMG and ENG characteristics of anterior horn cell disease may be summarised as follows:
  spontaneous activity dependent on acuteness of process;
  pronounced evidence of collateral sprouting; large amplitudes;
  usually normal conduction velocity.

*a) Generalised Anterior Horn Cell Diseases.* These include:
Progressive infantile spinal muscular atrophy (Werdnig-Hoffmann)
Proximal spinal muscular atrophy (Kugelberg-Welander)
Motor neurone disease in adults

- Aran–Duchenne type
- Vulpian–Bernhardt type
- Calf-thigh type (Bodechthel-Schrader)
- Progressive bulbar palsy
- Amyotrophic lateral sclerosis

EMG affords a means of early diagnosis of these generalised disorders; even though clinically the lesion may appear to be a localised one of a muscle or group of muscles, the EMG will reveal its generalised nature. Needle recording fron tongue and face muscles should help to differentiate bulbar palsy from pseudo-bulbar palsy.

The commonest of the above -mentioned group of diseases is amyotrophic lateral sclerosis, and this generally occurs in the elderly. Both the upper and the lower motor neurone are involved, though the clinical emphasis may fall on one or the other at first. As soon as anterior horn cells are affected the EMG will help to determine the nature of the hitherto perhaps entirely upper motor neurone lesion.

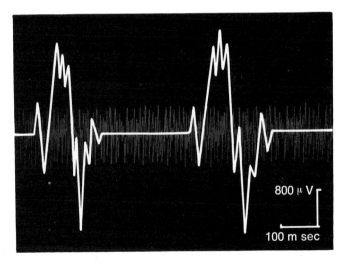

Fig. 16. Giant potential in anterior horn cell damage (see also Fig. 17 example of amyotrophic lateral sclerosis)

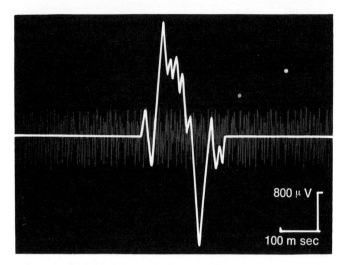

Fig. 17. So-called giant potential, distinguished by pronounced increase in amplitude and duration and by polyphasia; the result of peripheral sprouting and increase in motor unit territory. Note the smaller normal example (chronic poliomyelitis)

*b) Local Disorders of Anterior Horn Cells: Poliomyelitis.* The active disease is rarely seen today thanks to successful immunisation, but EMG may be helpful in the post-poliomyelitic state, thus:

The concentric needle may reveal spontaneous activity many years after infection, usually in the shape of fibrillation potentials. This raises the possibility that the infection may not, in fact, be quite dead, and a very slow progression would explain the occurrence of gradually diminishing motor function. A sudden deterioration of function following an apparently halted earlier infection may have a different explanation however. It may be that the normal physiological stresses and strains of life have just been sufficient to "decompensate" those motor units which have greatly enlarged their responsibilities through collateral sprouting and hence have a reduced reserve. The myasthenic reaction of such motor units to repetitive stimulation may represent such imminent failure of function. It is important that EMG be used to clearly delineate that musculature which remains intact or largely so, in order to reduce confusion at a later stage of clinical assessment.

## Syringomyelia

Here the EMG can demonstrate a neurogenic lesion with the characteristics of anterior horn cell damage, but having a segmental distribution. Chronic denervation is usually prominent, according to the state of progression of the disease, and its course may be followed electrophysiologically.

### 3.2.1.3. Root Lesions

*a) The Intervertebral Disc.* Here prolapse provides the commonest cause of root lesions. "Irritation" of the anterior root without actual fibre degeneration will result in segmentally-distributed fasciculation. When fibre loss has occurred, however, fibrillation potentials will appear early in monosegmentally-innervated paraspinal muscles, but only after 2–3 weeks in distal limb muscles. Usually two roots are involved, giving a myotomal picture.

An accurate determination of the distribution of peripheral abnormalities is essential in differential diagnosis, for example, between an L5 root lesion and a lateral popliteal nerve palsy. As in anterior horn cell disease, motor conduction velocity is normal.

When relapse follows operation for a prolapsed disc it may be difficult to decide whether the old lesion is responsible or a new segment is affected. Denervation may be due to the first lesion, if it is of relatively recent occurrence, as well as a new one, and EMG is therefore limited in its usefulness to documenting variations in the amount of denervation. Myelography is of course the appropriate investigation in cases of severe clinical relapse. It is helpful in assessing the likelihood of another segment having been affected to have the operation report. Paravertebral recording soon after operation may reveal denervation due only to local trauma.

*b) Cervical 'Whiplash' Injury.* This is observed in increasing numbers with the rise in traffic accidents. EMG may help to decide if a root injury has been caused, when fibrillation will appear after 2–3 weeks; fasciculation is less often met with. Again, paracervical recording will show denervation earlier, though such recordings are more difficult to make than in the case of extremity muscles. Medico-legal considerations make EMG advisable in all cases of whiplash injury.

c) *Polyradiculitis (Guillain-Barré)*. After 3–4 weeks EMG will usually provide objective evidence of this condition: fibrillation indicating recent denervation, and prolonged distal latencies.

d) *Other Varieties of Root Lesion*. Local bony abnormalities may result in root lesions which can be detected by paravertebral EMG studies.

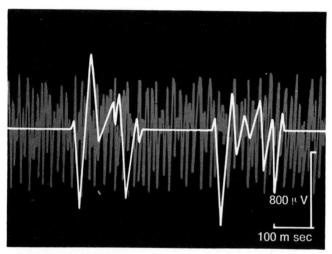

Fig. 18. Neurogenic reconstruction with two motor unit action potentials, clearly differentiated by increased duration, polyphasia and, less markedly, amplitude. (Example of a partial plexus lesion, which is difficult to distinguish from regenerative processes occurring in a local distal lesion; other criteria will have to be taken into account)

*3.2.1.4. Plexus Lesions*

EMG has an important part to play both in differentiating plexus from root lesions and in determining the precise part of the plexus affected. It has the advantage over clinical examination that the action of individual muscles will not be masked by synergy. No plexus injury can be considered properly evaluated without EMG, and in order of frequency such conditions are:
 Traumatic (including birth trauma)
 Neuralgic amyotrophy ("plexus neuritis")
 Plexus compression (e.g. by cervical rib)
 Post-mastectomy complications

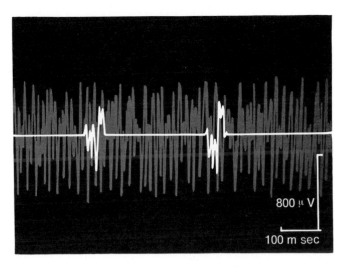

Fig. 21. Reinnervation potential in its later stages (example Fig. 20)

*Compressive Neuropathy*

EMG and ENG have revealed that local compression neuropathies are more frequent than had been supposed. It has, for example, been shown that patients with pain in the arm diagnosed as "brachialgia" – a nonspecific and vague term – must often have been suffering from carpal tunnel compression of the median nerve.

*a) Carpal Tunnel Syndrome.* A prolonged distal sensory or motor conduction time will reveal the presence of compression of the median nerve before there has been substantial fibre damage, and will differentiate the condition from a root syndrome by showing that abnormal findings are limited to the median distribution. Early diagnosis will facilitate effective treatment.

*b) Cubital Sulcus Syndrome.* The next most common lesion of this kind is the compression of the ulnar nerve which occurs at the elbow, sometimes occupational but, again, often apparently spontaneous. Before clear neurological deficit has occurred, the site and severity of the lesion may be determined by EMG and ENG. A deep lesion of the ulnar nerve at the wrist or in the hand also occurs and can be identified by the usual principles. The usual differential diagnosis in the case of an ulnar palsy is a root lesion (C8/T1) or system disease (e.g. motor neurone disease); compression palsy of this nerve is especially likely to occur in bedridden patients.

In each case of compressive neuropathy the question arises as to whether this is merely a local manifestation of a widespread but subclinical neuropathy. This consideration emphasises the importance of not restricting the investigation exclusively to the affected part: enough should be done to exclude possibilities such as polyneuropathy, even when the lesion seems obviously purely local.

*c) Radial Nerve.* Here we encounter the "Saturday night" or "park bench" palsy, a neurapraxia due to compression of the nerve in the spiral groove and having a favourable prognosis (see p. 35). A true chronic compression of the nerve does occur at the elbow in relation to the supinator muscle, when EMG, by facilitating early diagnosis, may prevent irreversible damage.

*d) Chronic Compressive Neuropathies of the Lower Limb.* These are less common than in the upper limb, but a lesion of the lateral popliteal nerve at the fibular head is apt to develop in bidridden patients, and may sometimes have to be distinguished from the tibialis anterior syndrome. The tarsal tunnel syndrome and Morton's metatarsalgia are diagnosed too rarely. Damage due to pressure from plaster casts, wire extensions and callus formation can occur, and be usefully investigated by means of EMG and ENG.

*Idiopathic Facial Nerve Palsy (Bell's)*

The facial nerve may be acutely damaged, by the pressure of oedema, where it lies in its rigid bony canal in the temporal bone. The damage may result in a fleeting conduction block, completely reversible (i.e. neurapraxia), or in fibre degeneration with the nerve in continuity (i.e. axonotmesis). Which of these forms of injury occurs is probably determined in the first few hours, so that operative decompression would be the management of choice if only clinical differentiation were possible. Even EMG is not immediately useful, since the nerve will continue to conduct impulses to the facial muscles when stimulated distal to the lesion (as it must be) until degeneration occurs after a few days, and fibrillation will not appear in the first week after injury. Stimulation of the nerve at this time may, however, show a distal motor latency of more than 4 msec, and experience has shown that this indicates denervation. By this time it is too late for surgery. Where denervation has

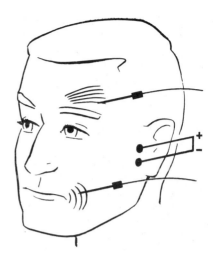

Fig. 22. Illustrating the usual stimulation and recording points for the facial nerve. Recordings from orbicularis oculi are possible in the same way when the needle is carefully inserted

occurred, reinnervation may be followed with the concentric needle during the subsequent 8–12 weeks. Once the first reinnervation potentials have appeared in denervated muscle further electrical therapy (if employed) is pointless, since it is impossible to prevent abnormal sprouting of the nerve. Should this occur, the development of faulty reinnervation and abnormal movements may be studied by means of ENG.

*Trigeminal Neuropathy*

The finding of denervation potentials in the temporal or masseter muscles will indicate that trigeminal neuralgia is symptomatic and not idiopathic.

*Polyneuropathies*

EMG and ENG may help to detect a polyneuropathy in an early, if not pre-clinical, stage, since weakness of a muscle does not become apparent until a certain proportion of motor fibres have degenerated. However, the first electrophysiological sign of a polyneuropathy may be a change in the sensory ENG. Since most polyneuropathies have a chronic progressive course, signs of chronic denervation may be to the forefront, while fibrillation and positive sharp waves may be infrequently met with. The most important single finding is that of increased distal conduction times; the first electrophysiological abnormal-

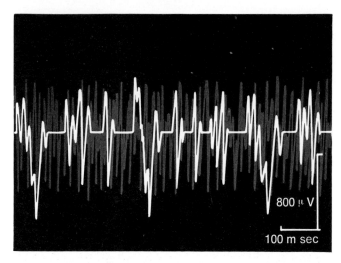

Fig. 23. Neurogenic reconstruction. Depicted are three reconstructed units with increased potential duration and polyphasia without any significant increase in amplitude. The interference pattern is hardly changed. Unimportant rarefaction (example of a distal polyneuropathy)

ity is apt to be manifest in the most distal parts of the nerve. The widespread finding of a reduced interference pattern is also of value in this diagnosis, but here a warning must be sounded: changes indistinguishable from a polyneuropathy may be detected with the EMG in the small foot muscles of the normal subject, so such findings would have to be supported by others, such as a prolonged distal latency, and findings in the upper limbs such as reduced sensory action potentials. If the process primarily affects the most peripheral nerve twigs, the fall-out of single muscle fibres or small groups may result in a pattern resembling the myopathic, at least initially and before sprouting has started to occur. Perhaps the same mechanism underlies the apparent neurogenic changes seen in certain muscular dystrophies of long standing. The only safe approach in this situation is to sample many different sites with the needle, so as to gain a more comprehensive picture. Then a firm statement should be possible, and vague and imprecise terms such as "neuromyopathy" avoided. The EMG and ENG are helpful in the investigation of so-called diabetic amyotrophy, which is actually a proximal motor neuropathy showing itself as pain, weakness and wasting of the quadriceps.

As already mentioned, the slowing of conduction in a nerve affected by a polyneuropathy may first show itself at a site at which it normally is subject to some stress or trauma. Biochemical investigations will here play their part in diagnosis.

*Peroneal Muscular Atrophy*

This disease of the nervous system is characterised by extreme slowing of nerve conduction, e.g. to 30m/sec or less, and by the EMG changes of polyneuropathic type.

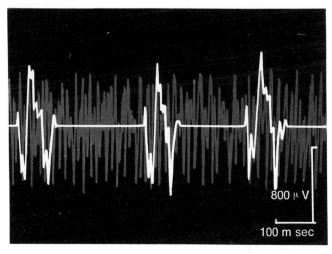

Fig. 24. Neurogenic reconstruction as a result of chronic denervation in the distal part of the lower motor neurone with obvious rarefaction (example of a neural muscle atrophy)

### 3.2.2. Primary Muscle Disease

Since pathological changes in muscle disease are often, initially at any rate, of patchy distribution, the muscle should be sampled systematically at as many sites as is practicable. As already mentioned, the changes characteristic of myopathy are common to this whole group of disorders, and do not provide nosological diagnoses in individual cases. Muscle biopsy is an essential complementary investigation, and is generally performed after EMG, though not, of course, on a muscle which has been recently sampled with a needle.

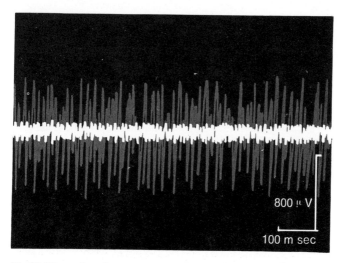

Fig. 25. Illustration of myopathy. Distinct reduction in amplitude, polyphasia and reduced mean action potential duration; (example of Duchenne dystrophy in early stage)

### 3.2.2.1. Progressive Muscular Dystrophy (Duchenne)

Early in the disease spontaneous activity is not evident and, owing to early recruitment, an interference pattern is present. Individual motor unit action potential duration is reduced (1–3 msec), and amplitudes are generally down to 300–800 µV. In advanced stages spontaneous activity may occasionally be seen, and is attributable to a reduction in muscle membrane potential. Areas of fat deposition may give a picture on needle sampling of "silent areas", in clear contrast to the adjacent pseudohypertrophic muscle.

### 3.2.2.2. Inflammatory Muscle Disease (Myositis and Polymyositis)

In contrast to the degenerative primary muscle diseases, inflammation usually leads to early fibre drop-out and spontaneous activity in the form of fibrillation potentials occurring in short bursts here and there. Early recruiting may also be seen, potential duration is shortened (1–4 msec), and amplitude reduced (60–100 µV). Polyphasia is prominent. EMG is an indispensable method of following the course of the disease and the response to treatment.

## 3.2.2.3. Late-Onset Myopathies

Elderly invalids, especially women, with proximal weakness may on examination be found to have a true myopathy.

## 3.2.2.4. Hereditary Distal Myopathy (Welander)

By means of EMG and ENG it is possible to distinguish this very rare form of myopathy from a polyneuropathy.

## 3.2.2.5. Myotonia

There is an hyperirritability of muscle in true myotonia, so that percussion of the muscle results in a visible knot appearing transiently, and a needle in such muscle shows spontaneous discharges of high but falling frequency and amplitude. (more than 100/sec sometimes). Acoustically these discharges sound like a "dive-bomber". Such a myotonic reaction appears on needle insertion, needle movement and removal, percussion of the muscle, and both during and after voluntary activation. The last do not necessarily show the typical waxing and waning. The pattern of recruitment on voluntary activation does not change. The features described may occur in dystrophia myotonica, and also in the hyperkalaemic form of periodic paralysis. Since myotonia often precedes dystrophy, the finding of a myotonic reaction can be of diagnostic value early in the course of dystrophia myotonica.
In other disorders of nerve and muscle high frequency discharges of bizarrely shaped potentials are not infrequently seen, but these start

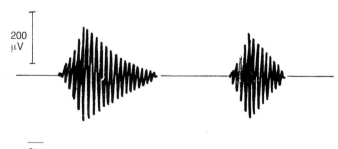

Fig. 26. Myotonic discharges

and stop suddenly and do not show the above-mentioned fluctuation in frequency and amplitude. They are sometimes referred to as "pseudo-myotonic discharges".

### 3.2.3. Secondary Myopathies

In the case of the myopathy which may form part of an endocrine, metabolic or toxic disorder, important clues may be provided by the EMG before clinical weakness is manifest. Disuse atrophy may, but usually does not, show changes of myopathic kind.

### 3.2.4. Myasthenic Syndromes

*3.2.4.1. Myasthenia Gravis*

The diagnosis of myasthenia gravis is probable when a decrement in amplitude of a third occurs in the course of repetitive stimulation at less than 25/sec. If a parenteral dose of Tensilon reverses this reduction in amplitude, the diagnosis is almost certain.

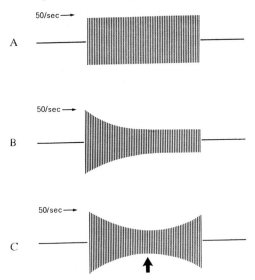

Fig. 27. The myasthenic reaction.
Repetitive stimulation at 50/sec: A No amplitude reduction in normal subjects, B Clear reduction by over $1/3$ in myasthenia gravis, C Abolishing the reduction with I. V. Tensilon

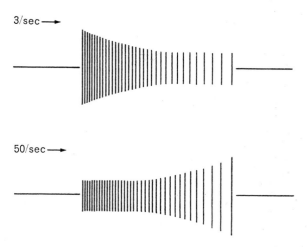

Fig. 28. The response to repetitive stimulation in the Eaton-Lambert syndrome (see text)

### 3.2.4.2. Symptomatic Myasthenia

This may occur in cases of polymyositis, when the primary diagnosis will be indicated by the changes already described in this type of disorder. The Tensilon test is negative or weakly positive. Rarely an actual increase in amplitude occurs. The rare but important accompaniment of certain bronchial carcinomas, the *Eaton-Lambert* syndrome, has certain unique electrophysiological features which help to distinguish it from myasthenia gravis, namely:
1. An *increase* in amplitude of the response to supramaximal stimulation at frequencies of over 40/sec (facilitation), but the usual decrease at 1–3/sec, as in true myasthenia.
2. Little or no response to Tensilon.

### 3.2.5. Electrolyte Disturbances

By means of certain provocative measures (see p. 27) the EMG may reveal a latent tetany: multiple discharges are seen. The motor unit activity of carpo-pedal spasm may confuse the issue, and recording multiple discharges is best done after provocation has ended. Repetitive multiple discharges may also be observed in hypocalcaemia, while hyperkalaemia, by contrast, may be accompnied by myotonia. Valuable information may be gained from ENG in the course of the electrolyte

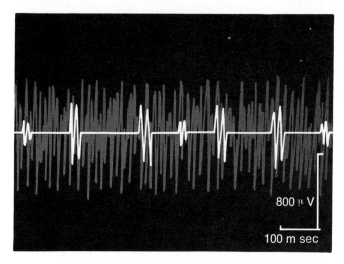

Fig. 29. Repetitive discharge of two so-called doublets (tetany)

disturbances accompanying chronic renal insufficiency, dialysis, or after renal transplant.

### 3.2.6. Myxoedema

In myxoedema there is a prolonged relaxation time when a deep tendon reflex (e.g. Achilles) is elicited, and this can be quantitated by means of mechanographic equipment.

### 3.2.7. Tetanus

The EMG can be of decisive importance in the early diagnosis of this condition. The smallest of voluntary movements, pain, even a loud noise, may result in prolonged spasm of skeletal musculature, which can be recorded with the EMG. An example is trismus. There may also be a shortened or absent "silent period".

### 3.2.8. Centrally-Determined Disturbances of Movement

Exact quantitative analysis of these problems necessitates a multiple channel electromyograph, so only those clinical conditions will be discussed which can be investigated by means of a single channel machine.

*3.2.8.1. Spasticity*

Even when spasticity is still clinically latent it may be possible with the EMG to demonstrate increased reflex excitability. Spontaneous activity in relaxed muscles is, of course, absent. Passive extension causes reflexly-induced spastic contractions, characterised electromyographically by relatively slow discharge of individual motor units. Clinically latent spasticity may also be revealed by means of the injection of 5 mgm succinylcholine.

*3.2.8.2. Rigidity*

In contrast to spasticity, motor unit activity is present in rigidity even in the apparently relaxed muscle, and the potentials show a tendency to grouping. On passive extension there is an initial increase in this background activity, which is suppressed by extension beyond a certain point. A slight contraction will then cause a rapid reappearance of the background activity. This is known as the release phenomenon.

*3.2.8.3. Tremor*

*a) Rest Tremor in Extrapyramidal Disease.* Here there is a tremor at rest which is partly or wholly suppressed by voluntary movement of the affected limb(s). The EMG shows groups of motor unit action potentials recurring regularly at the tremor rate, usually 4–8/sec. The pattern may vary from examination to examination in the same patient. A needle in the antagonists will show similar grouped discharges alternating with those of the agonists.

*b) Intention Tremor.* EMG recording in intention tremor is difficult owing to inevitable movement artefact. It is not, in any case, of particular value.

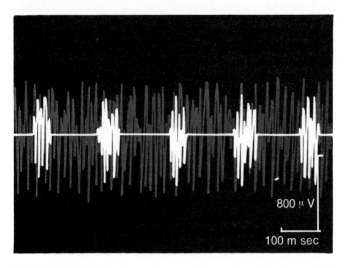

Fig. 30. Rhythmical discharge of a group of normal motor unit potentials as an expression of a quiet tremor (Parkinson's disease)

### 3.2.8.4. Torticollis

Predominantly tonic and predominantly clonic forms may be differentiated electromyographically. The first is characterised by continuous background activity, the second by grouped discharges. There is synergy between the sternomastoid on one side and deep neck muscles on the other, so recording should be made simultaneously in the former muscle and in splenius capitis.

### 3.2.9. EMG, ENG and the "Floppy Infant" Syndrome

The EMG has proved of great value in the assessment and differential diagnosis of the rather heterogeneous collection of disorders which give rise to this syndrome. Sampling with a needle electrode can, for obvious reasons, be difficult in this age group, since spontaneous activity may be masked by movement and motor unit activity may have to be evoked by means of reflexes. It is nevertheless generally possible to differentiate central, peripheral neurogenic and myopathic disorders, though the detection of myasthenia presents much greater problems.

### 3.2.9.1. Peripheral Neurogenic Lesions

Here one is mainly concerned with the recognition of infantile spinal muscular atrophy. As in the anterior horn cell diseases of maturity, large, polyphasic units and fasciculation (often not visible through the skin because of the childs fat) are prominent.
In metachromatic leucodystrophy the extreme slowing of motor conduction velocity – to 20 m/sec or less (see also p. 20) – is of cardinal importance in diagnosis.
In arthrogryposis multiplex congenita the abnormality may be confined to rarefaction of the pattern on maximal voluntary effort. There is assumed to be an hereditarily-determined deficiency in the anterior horn cells, the surviving ones discharging at an increased frequency.

### 3.2.9.2. Myogenic Pareses

Infantile muscular dystrophy may be identified if the EMG signs of a myopathy are present, but the systematic sampling recommended earlier is not usually possible in the very young and a biopsy may be necessary.

### 3.2.9.3. Centrally-Determined Disturbances of Movement

Qualitative changes are naturally absent from the EMG and ENG in supranuclear lesions, but by exclusion of peripheral neurogenic or myogenic lesions the clinical diagnosis may be confirmed. The distinction from benign muscular hypotonia is not possible, because here also qualitative changes are absent.

## 4.0. EMG of the Extraocular Muscles

It is often of great importance to decide whether an impairment of eye movement is the result of a myopathy, a neurogenic lesion, myasthenia, or a central disturbance. Sampling with a concentric needle electrode may provide the answer, and EMG of these muscles has the following characteristics:

1. Since the extraocular muscles have very small motor units the appearance of both individual motor unit action potentials and the pattern on activity is different from that in skeletal musculature. Potentials are of shorter duration and discharge frequencies are higher.

2. In contrast to relaxed skeletal muscle, eye muscle, even in the neutral position of the globe, shows constant activity. Even when antagonists are maximally active, agonists will show motor unit activity.

## 4.1. Myopathies

*a) Oligo-Symptomatic Form of Ocular Myositis.* From the early beginnings of EMG as a diagnostic tool it has been possible to show that weakness of extraocular muscles is often the result of a myositis. In the chronic forms, signs of inflammation may be minimal or absent, and pain on movement admitted only on direct questioning. EMG, therefore, is of great importance, since timely treatment with corticosteroids is then possible.

It is not easy to be sure that a myopathy is present in these muscles as the potentials are very short even in normal subjects. The inflammatory process involves almost all muscles, however, while muscles supplied by cranial nerves are generally easily identified. Since a reduction in amplitude and a shortening of potential duration do not help here in the diagnosis, the criterion of early recruitment is correspondingly more important. With myogenic paresis a complete interference pattern is found even when eye movement is barely recognisable clinically.

*b) Acute Exophthalmic Myositis.* Acute ocular myositis with exophthalmos must be differentiated from a retro-orbital tumour. This is usually possible with EMG, and therapy with steroids may be started.

*c) Ocular Muscle Dystrophy.* The ocular form of a chronic muscular dystrophy manifests itself first in the elevators. The EMG may show that clinically unsuspected involvement of shoulder girdle muscles is present, and in fact the extraocular muscles are rarely attacked alone in this condition.

*d) Endocrine Ocular Myopathy.* Again, the elevators are the most frequently involved, and the EMG pattern is that of a myopathy as a rule.

*e) Ocular Myotonia.* In dystrophia myotonica, as well as in Thomsen's disease, the extraocular muscles are seldom attacked, but their occasional involvement may be demonstrated with the EMG.

*f) Ocular Myasthenia.* The clinical differentiation of ocular myasthenia from oligo-symptomatic myositis is difficult and only EMG is really helpful. Characteristically the frequency and amplitude of individual motor unit action potentials fall off during voluntary effort, through gradual drop-out of motor units. This may be demonstrated by means of the Tensilon test: a few seconds after IV injection of 5–10 mgm Tensilon there is a significant increase in activity, usually an interference pattern, but the effect is short-lived.

## 4.2. Peripheral Neurogenic Paresis

Here one is mainly concerned with the effects of trauma. Differentiation may be made electromyographically between primary nerve injury and a "strangulation" of the muscle by orbital fracture, since in the former there will be signs of denervation; again, the very shortness of normal potentials in these muscles renders them liable to confusion with denervation potentials.

## 4.3. Centrally-Determined Disturbances of Movement

Qualitative changes are here absent from the EMG. Paradoxical innervation such as in Duane's syndrome may be found, but simultaneous recordings are advisable as proof. EMG help is especially valuable before surgery.

## 5.0. Possibilities of Error in the EMG

Artefacts are of less importance than in other electrodiagnostic techniques, but may be considered under two headings:

1. Artefacts in the narrow sense of the word, due to disturbances originating outside the musculature being examined. Special screening measures are not required as a rule, though AC hum and other electrical activity sometimes upsets the recording. A correctly positioned earth electrode will usually prevent this kind of trouble.

2. Phenomena associated with sampling with the concentric needle electrode, but which are physiological, such as endplate noise, which may be mistaken for spontaneous activity of pathological type. Repositioning the needle will quickly abolish endplate noise, while fibrillation is apt to be increased by needle movement. Potential changes due to deficient electrical contacts or poorly polarised needles may arise independently of apparent needle movement, and may cause confusion with motor unit activity.

Misinterpretations based on insufficient relaxation of the patient can be avoided if one considers individual findings only in the context of the whole picture.

## 5.1. Possibilities of Error in the ENG

*a) Motor Electroneurogram.* Even with proper technique, errors are possible. For example, the exact moment of take-off from the baseline is sometimes open to discussion. Supramaximal stimulation is not always achieved, and latencies may seem to be longer than they are.

*b) Sensory Electroneurogram.* The above considerations apply also to the sensory ENG, but in addition one should pay attention to details such as correct placement of electrodes, reduction of skin resistance, proper choice of filters and so on.
In both situations latencies must measured be as accurately as possible.

# 6.0. Short Introduction to an EMG Examination

1. Preparation. The object and form of the investigation is explained to the patient, and he is instructed as to how he may best co-operate. Weak and full effort with those muscles which will be examined are rehearsed without needles. The patient is then brought to a relaxed state in a comfortable position.

2. The earth electrode is attached to the extremity in which the investigation will start.

3. The machine is switched on, with the gain control set at high amplification so that spontaneous activity will not be missed.

4. Cleaning of the skin at the intended point of insertion. The needle should be placed rapidly and cleanly into the muscle, without fuss, and the machine set ready to pick up the earliest activity.

5. The screen is watched for several minutes to see if spontaneous activity occurs, the needle position being changed several times in a vertical direction.

6. The form and duration of motor unit potentials on weak voluntary effort are noted.

7. On maximal voluntary effort it is noted whether the pattern is of full interference or is rarefied to any degree; on moderate effort the recruiting pattern can be observed.

8. When the patient is asked to relax after maximal voluntary effort it should be noted whether activity comes to an abrupt end, or whether there is some after-discharge as in myotonia.

9. When recording from small muscles of the hands and feet distal motor latencies are always measured in affected muscles.

10. The needle is rapidly removed.

11. Short notes are made concerning the findings in each muscle examined.

The EMG examination may be considered concluded when the examiner has gained an adequate impression of the state of function and is able to answer the necessary clinical questions. His ability to do this will depend on the number of muscles examined and the extent to which they have been explored.

## 7.0. Index of Important Terms in Clinical EMG

*Artefact:* Technical artefacts which originate within or without the machine are different from those which originate in the muscle being examined. On the whole, artefacts do not play a large part in electromyography.

*Doublets and Triplets:* Rhythmic multiple discharges which indicate a disturbance of electrolyte metabolism. They mostly appear only on suitable provocation.

*Endplate Noise:* Repetitive discharge of low voltage potentials which appear when the point of the needle lies near the endplate zone. Differentiation from true spontaneous activity is possible by changing the position of the needle.

*Discharge Frequency:* The frequency with which a motor unit "fires" during the examination.

*Fasciculation Potentials:* The bioelectrical correlate of the involuntary activity of whole motor units; an expression of hyperirritability of the lower motor neurone which may be benign or malignant and which are most commonly seen in anterior horn cell and root lesions.

*Fibrillation Potentials And Positive Sharp Waves:* The bioelectrical correlates of individual muscle fibre contractions. Physiologically, fibres contract only in the context of the whole motor unit, so fibrillation expresses functional discontinuity between nerve fibre and muscle fibre. They are most commonly found in denervation processes (Wallerian degeneration), but may also occur in long standing dystrophies and acute myositis.

*High Frequency Discharges:* "Pseudo-myotonic" discharges which occur in a variety of conditions and which differ from true myotonia in their sudden onset and end, and in their relatively constant amplitude and frequency.

*Insertion Activity:* Low voltage, fleeting discharges which occur only momentarily on needle insertion and may therefore be heard rather than seen. Their exact origin is not known, but their absence from necrotic or completely denervated muscle is of importance.

*Interference pattern:* The pattern of activity seen during full effort by a healthy muscle, in which no base line is seen because potentials are all interfering with one another.

*Latency:* The time interval between stimulus and first deflection of the muscle action potential from the base-line. The distal latency is of particular importance clinically.

*Myasthenic Reaction:* A pathological fall-off in amplitude and dropout of motor units during repetitive stimulation: an expression of endplate dysfunction. In the Eaton-Lambert syndrome (paraneoplastic myasthenia) facilitation occurs at fast stimulation frequencies, and the response to Tensilon is small or absent. Both these points differentiate it from myasthenia gravis.

*Motor Unit Action Potential:* The bioelectrical correlate of the motor unit (Sherrington). Its form and duration depend primarily upon the number and spatial distribution of its constituent muscle fibres.

*Myotonic Reaction:* A high frequency discharge of potentials with a fluctuating amplitude and frequency occurring on needle insertion, percussion of the muscle or spontaneously.

*Neurogenic Reconstruction:* This occurs during chronic denervation processes, when peripheral sprouting of nerve terminals, or more proximal collateral sprouting, leads to a change in form and duration of the motor unit action potential. This includes the development of a larger than normal incidence of polyphasic potentials, and the enlargement of motor unit territory.

*Positive Sharp Waves:* See Fibrillation potentials.

*Potential Duration:* The time in msec between the first deflection of a motor unit action potential from the base-line and its final return to it.

*Recruiting:* The order and manner in which individual motor units are activated during voluntary innervation. Early recruiting may indicate a myopathic process.

*Spontaneous Activity:* The appearance of action potentials in a relaxed muscle. Usually pathological. Three main types are: fibrillation, positive sharp waves and fasciculation (see under appropriate headings).

*Triplets:* See Doublets

## 8.0. Index of Important Technical Terms and Abbreviations

*Anode:* Electrode through which the main current exits from a system.

*Bandwidth:* The frequency interval of the amplifier being used.

*Hum:* Alternating current interference (at 50 or 60 Hz).

*Input Circuit:* Has the job of fitting the signal picked up at the source optimally to the amplifier.

*Input Capacity:* Determines the highest frequency which can be of practical use. The components and circuit capacity determine the unavoidable minimum input capacity.

*Input Resistance:* Its height limits the permissible source resistance (i.e. at the electrode). In order to be able to follow signal changes of less than 1% it should be over 100 times larger than the source resistance.

*Electrode:* a) of tubes: The structural element that conducts current (cathode, grid, anode); b) in diagnosis: Collector electrode for measuring potential differences; c) in therapy: Current contact used in coupling of stimulation currents on patients.

*Frequencies:* Number of cycles per second. Unit of measure: Hertz (Hz).

*Generator:* Electric device for generating voltage. A general term for power source.

*Impedance:* Total resistance: sum of ohmic and capacitive resistance.

*Cathode:* Electrode in the tube at which the current enters the discharge space.

*Oscillograph Tube:* Electron-ray tube for the visible representation of the time slope of electric signals.

*Noise:* Static fluctuation of the electron current in tubes and transistors, which can lead to disturbing interferences in the information signal.

*Transistor:* Term for the structural element consisting of an active semiconductor with at least three contacts, of which the one for the controlling- and that for the controlled circuit are common.

*X-Axis:* The axis of reference in a graphic representation; when using Cartesian coordinates, this is also called the abscissa. In electron-ray oscillographs it represents the time axis or time basis.

*Y-Axis:* The axis perpendicular (vertical) of the X-axis, also known as the ordinate. In oscillograph tubes it is the axis for measuring voltage.

$\mu V$ = micro volt = 1/10000 volt,
$nV$ = milli volt = 1/1000 volt,
msec = milli second = 1/1000 second,
c/s = cycle/second = Hz.

## 9.0. Selected Bibliography

BASMAJIAN, J.V.: Muscles Alive: Their Functions Revealed by Electromyography. 2nd ed. Baltimore: William & Wilkins 1968.
BUCHTHAL, F.: Einführung in die Elektromyographie. München-Berlin: Urban & Schwarzenberg 1958.
COHEN, H.L., BRUMLIK, J.: A Manual of Electromyography. New York-Evanston-London: Harper & Row 1969.
DRECHSLER, B.: Elektromyographie. Berlin: Verlag für Volk u. Gesundheit 1964.
ESSLEN, E., MAGUN, R.: Elektromyographie. Grundlagen und klinische Anwendung. Fortschr. Neurol. Psychiat. **26**, 153–199 (1958).
FULLERTON, P.M.: Peripheral nerve conduction in: Peripheral nerve conduction in metachromatic leucodystrophy (sulphatide lipidosis). J. Neurol. Neurosurg. Psychiat. **27**, 100–105 (1964).
GILLIATT, R.W., GOODMAN, H.V., WILLISON, R.G.: The recording of lateral popliteal nerve action potentials in man. J. Neurol. Neurosurg. Psychiat. **24**, 305–318 (1961).
HOPF, H.Ch.: Das Elektromyogramm bei Nervenreizung. Fortsch. Neurol. Psychiat., **31**, 585 (1963).
KAESER, H.E.: Die Elektromyographie als neurologische Hilfsmethode. Schweiz. Arch. Neurol. Neurochir. Psychiat. **101**, 11–30 (1968).
LENMAN, J.A.R., RITCHIE, A.E.: Clinical Electromyography. Pitman Press, Bath, 1970.
LICHT, G.: Electrodiagnosis and Electromyography. New Haven/CT: E. LICHT Publ. 1961.
MCCOMAS, A.J., MROZEK, K.: The electrical properties of muscle fibre membranes in dystrophia myotonica and myotonia congenita. J. Neurol. Neurosurg. Psychiat. **31**, 441–447 (1968).
STEINBRECHER, W.: Elektromyographie in Klinik und Praxis. Stuttgart: Thieme 1965.
STRUPPLER, A., RUPRECHT, E.O.: Elektromyographie (EMG) und Elektroneurographie (ENG). Grundlagen und diagnostische Bedeutung. Z.EEG-EMG **2**, 2–16 (1971).
STRUPPLER, A.: Klinische Elektromyographie. In: Hdb. d. Kinderheilkunde. Bd. 8, T. 1. Berlin-Heidelberg-New York: Springer 1969.
TROJABORG, W., BUCHTHAL, F.: Malignant and benign fasciculations. Acta Neurol. scand. **41**, suppl. 13, 251–254 (1965).
WYNN PARRY, C.B.: Techniques of neuromuscular stimulation and their clinical application. In: Disorders of Voluntary Muscle. (Ed. J.N. WALTON) London: Churchill 1964.

# 10.0. Subject Index

action potential, evoked muscle   19
–, motor unit   25
–, nerve and sensory   4
–, orthodromic   21
–, sensory   21
activity, insertion   15
–, spontaneous   15
–, voluntary   15
anterior horn cell diseases   30
artefact stimulus   19
artefacts   52
averager   9
–, digital   9
axonotmesis   35

Bell's palsy   38
belly-tendon   4
biopsy, muscle   41

"chronaxie"   4
collateral sprouting   30, 35
compressive neuropathy   37
conduction velocity   2, 19
– –, motor   49
– –, sensory   21
contractions, spastic   47

degeneration, Wallerian   23
delay line   9
denervation, chronic   33, 39
"denervation potential"   24
digital averager   9
discharge frequency   25
discharge, high frequency   24, 43
discharges, multiple   45
–, "pseudo-myotonic"   44
–, repetitive multiple   45
distal conduction, increased times   39
distal sensory latencies   22
disturbances, centrally-determined movement   27
–, metabolic electrolyte   27
– of movement, centrally-determined   47

electrodes   9–12
electrolyte, metabolic disturbances   27
electromyogram, normal   13
–, pathological   23

electromyograph, multiple channel   47
electroneurogram, motor   17
–, normal   17
–, pathological   27
–, sensory   20
EMG amplifier   7
EMG, extraocular muscles   49
end-plate noise   15
evoked muscle action potentials   4
extraocular muscles, EMG   49

facilitation   45
fasciculation, "benign"   23
–, "malign"   23
– potential   23
fibrillation   39
– potential   24, 42
firing rate   15
"floppy infant" syndrome   48
frequency, discharge   25
F wave   5

"giant potentials"   30

H wave   5

idiopathic facial nerve palsy   38
"innervation ratio"   1
"interference pattern"   15
– –, normal   29

latencies, distal sensory   22
latency   19
leucodystrophy, metachromatic   49

metachromatic leucodystrophy   49
motor conduction velocity   49
motor electroneurogram   17
motor unit   1
– – "territory"   16
muscle action potential   2
muscle biopsy   41
muscle disease, primary   41
myasthenia gravis   28, 44
myasthenia, symptomatic   45
myotonic reaction   43

nerve and sensory action potentials   4

neurapraxia  35
neuronotmesis  35
neuropathy, compressive  37
–, trigeminal  39
noise, end-plate  15

orthodromic action potential  21

palsy, idiopathic facial nerve  38
paravertebral recording  33
polyneuropathies  39
polyphasic potential  16
positive sharp waves  39
potential, "denervation"  24
–, evoked muscle action  4, 19
–, fasciculation  23
–, fibrillation  24, 42
–, "giant"  30
–, motor unit action  25
–, muscle action  2
–, orthodromic action  21
–, polyphasic  16
–, reflex  5
–, reinnervation  39
"pseudo-myotonic discharges"  44

reaction, myotonic  43

recording, extracellular  13
–, paravertebral  33
reflex potentials  5
"refractory period"  3
reinnervation  35, 36
release phenomenon  47
repetitive multiple discharges  45
repetitive stimulation  23, 44
root lesions  33

sensory action potential  21
"silent areas"  42
"silent period"  46
spastic contractions  47
sprouting, collateral  30
stimulation  3
–, repetitive  23, 44
–, supramaximal  3, 52
stimulus artefact  19
symptomatic myasthenia  45

Tensilon test  45
trigeminal neuropathy  39

Wallerian degeneration  23
waves, positive sharp  24

**T. Nomura**
**Atlas of Cerebral Angiography**

24 figures. 1 color plate
212 special plates, 6 angiograms
XI, 322 pages. 1970
ISBN 3-540-05222-4
Cloth DM 90,–
ISBN 0-387-05222-4
Cloth US $31.00

Published by Igaku Shoin Ltd., Tokyo. Sole distribution rights in all countries except the Far East: Springer-Verlag

**Cerebral Blood Flow**
Clinical and Experimental Results

Editors: M. Brock, C. Fieschi, D.H. Ingvar, N.A. Lassen, K. Schürmann
113 figures. XX, 291 pages. 1969
ISBN 3-540-04436-1
Cloth DM 68,–
ISBN 0-387-04436-1
Cloth US $18.40

**Cerebral Circulation and Metabolism**
6th International Symposium

Editor: M. Reivich
216 figures. 82 tables.
Approx. 530 pages. 1974
In preparation.
ISBN 3-540-06645-4

Distribution rights for Japan: Nankodo Co. Ltd., Tokyo

**J.F. Kurtzke**
**Epidemiology of Cerebrovascular Disease**

42 figures. XV, 197 pages. 1969
ISBN 3-540-04591-0
Cloth DM 74,–
ISBN 0-387-04591-0
Cloth US $30.20

**Handbook of Sensory Physiology**

Editorial Board: H. Autrum, R. Jung, W.R. Loewenstein, D.M. MacKay, H.L. Teuber
In 9 volumes
Please ask for information

**Intracranial Pressure**
Experimental and Clinical Aspects

Editors: M. Brock, H. Dietz
142 figures. XVI, 383 pages. 1972
ISBN 3-540-06039-1
Cloth DM 78,–
ISBN 0-387-06039-1
Cloth US $29.30

**A. Mostafawy**
**Pediatric Sonoencephalography**
The Practical Use of Ultrasonic Echoes in the Diagnosis of Childhood Intracranial Disorders

In Cooperation with J.B. Nagle
52 figures. XI, 137 pages. 1971
ISBN 3-540-05216-X
Cloth DM 86,–
ISBN 0-387-05216-X
Cloth US $30.10

Prices are subject to change without notice

**Springer-Verlag**
**Berlin**
**Heidelberg**
**New York**

## Radiological Exploration of the Ventricles and Subarachnoid Space

By G. Ruggiero, J. Bories, A. Calabrò, G. Cristi, G. Scialfa, F. Smaltino, A. Thibaut
With the cooperation of G. Gianasi, G. Maranghi, C. Philippart, E. Signorini
90 partly colored figures (279 sparate illustrations)
XIV, 152 pages. 1974

ISBN 3-540-06572-5
Cloth DM 148,—
ISBN 0-387-06572-5
Cloth US $60.40

Distribution rights for Japan: Igaku Shoin Ltd., Tokyo

## M. Wiesendanger
## Pathophysiology of Muscle Tone

4 figures. V, 46 pages. 1972
(Schriftenreihe Neurologie, Band 9).

ISBN 3-540-05761-7
Cloth DM 31,—
ISBN 0-387-05761-7
Cloth US $10.80

Prices are subject to change without notice

# Springer-Verlag
# Berlin
# Heidelberg
# New York

# Zeitschriften

## Journal of Neurology / Zeitschrift für Neurologie

Organ of the Deutsche Gesellschaft für Neurologie and the Deutsche Gesellschaft für Neurochirurgie

Editorial Board: M. Alter, H. Bauer, C. Fazio, E.J. Field, J.A. Kappers, F. Lhermitte, A. Lowenthal, M. Mumenthaler (Editor-in-Chief) S. Refsum, H. Reisner, G. Schaltenbrand, K. Schürmann, W. Tönnis, K.J. Zülch
1975, Vols. 209-210 (4 issues each): DM 336,—;
approx. US $137.10
plus postage and handling

## Neuroradiology

Organ of the European Society of Neuroradiology. Editorial Board: P. Amundsen, N. Azambuja, J. Bories, J.W.D. Bull, R. Chrzanowski, G. Cornelis, S. Cronqvist, D.O. Davies, G. Di Chiro, R. Djindjian, R. Ethier, K. Hara, P. Huber, J. Jirout, E.M. Klausberger, G. Lombardi, T.H. Newton, G. Ruggiero, M.M. Schechter (Editorial Secretary), J. Solé Llenas M. Takahashi, J. Taveras, A. Wackenheim (Editorial Secretary), S. Wende (Editorial Secretary), B.G. Ziedses des Plantes, L.H. Zingesser
1975, Vols. 9-10 (5 issues each): DM 232,—; approx. US $94.70
plus postage and handling